The Use of Counselling Skills
A Guide for Therapists

Skills for Practice Series

Series editors: Sally French and Jo Laing

Titles published

In preparation

• Skills for Practice •

The Use of Counselling Skills
A Guide for Therapists

John Swain
BSc, PGCE, MSc, PhD
Senior Lecturer,
Faculty of Health, Social Work and Education,
University of Northumbria

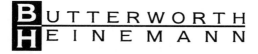

Butterworth-Heinemann Ltd
Linacre House, Jordan Hill, Oxford OX2 8DP

A member of the Reed Elsevier plc group

OXFORD   LONDON   BOSTON
MUNICH   NEW DELHI   SINGAPORE   SYDNEY
TOKYO   TORONTO   WELLINGTON

First edition 1995

© Butterworth-Heinemann Ltd 1995

British Library Cataloguing in Publication Data
A catalogue record for this book is available from the British Library

ISBN 0 7506 1618 0

Library of Congress Cataloguing in Publication Data
A catalogue record for this book is available from the Library of Congress

Set by TecSet
Printed by Biddles, Guildford and Kings Lynn

Contents

Preface

This is a book of personal and professional exploration and reflection. It is not about your specific expertise in providing, or training to provide, a specific form of therapy: physiotherapy, occupational or speech and language therapy. Nor is it about a clearly defined set of skills that you supposedly do not have and must add to your repertoire to be an effective therapist. This book explores therapy as a process of people working together as people, rather than therapist, client, colleague and so on. It is about people's awareness of themselves and others in therapy, the processes of communication they engage in and their relationships in providing and receiving help. It is about, to capture it in a single phrase, the human relations of helping in therapy.

This is a book for therapists who share my view that the human relations of helping are crucial to therapeutic encounters. It aims to facilitate them in reflecting on the expertise they already have in self-awareness and communicating with and relating to others. In doing so, it does not act as a cookbook to offer recipes for good practice, but rather raises challenges and dilemmas for which there are no readily available, off-the-shelf solutions. The challenges not only come from therapists examining and developing their work and roles: they also emanate from clients. The growth of the Disability Movement has, for instance, challenged beliefs about the nature of 'disability' and the control of help. This is designed, then, as a book for you to use to your own ends in developing your practice in helping as a therapist through exploring the difficult questions which can arise in the use of counselling skills.

There are many people I would like to thank for all the help I have been given in all the thought, work, writing, heart-searching and production that went into this book. THANK YOU:

To Jade Swain, Sue Raine, Elaine Grayson, Bob Fordham, Sarah Donoghue and Carole Thirlaway for all their encouragement and thought-provoking suggestions.

To Jo Laing for helping me weed out some of the worst examples of poor expression.

To all the students I have worked with over the years who, if they read this book, will see that I listened and learnt much from them.

The poem 'Disability' by Jenni Meredith from *Mustn't Grumble: Writing by Disabled Women* edited by Lois Keith, first published by The Women's Press Ltd, 1994, 43 Great Sutton Street, London EC1V 0DX, reprinted on page 204 is used by permission of The Women's Press Ltd.

The untitled poem, page 84, by R.D. Laing from *Knots*, first published by Tavistock Publications, 1970, 11 New Fetter Lane, London EC4P 4EE, reprinted on page 183 is used by permission of Tavistock Publications.

Finally I would like to thank Sally French because she first suggested that I should write this book and her belief in me never seemed to waver.

John Swain

Dedication

To Anna, Daniel, Sam and Tamsin Swain

Introduction

What is this book about?

This book is about people, their feelings, thoughts and desires. It is also about those subtle and complex processes that connect people: communications; awareness of themselves and each other; and personal relationships. The overall intention of the book is to support therapists in constructing open and non-hierarchical relationships for shared decision-making, effective working partnerships and mutual empowerment. In working towards this, the book offers therapists a basis for: deepening and extending their knowledge of human relations; reviewing and developing the range of skills at their disposal in interpersonal encounters; and reflecting on their practice within this context.

Though it draws on the theory and techniques of counselling, this book is *not* about being an expert counsellor. It is about the expertise all therapists require when they offer or are asked for help, particularly in responding to the needs and requirements of clients as defined by clients themselves. A distinction can be made between (a) counselling in the formal sense of what counsellors do in their professional capacity, and (b) what is sometimes referred to as 'use of counselling skills' in the more *ad hoc* sense of being part of the work of all carers and helpers, professional and informal. What they have in common is, according to Bond (1993): respect for the other person's values, personal resources and capacity for self-determination. For therapists this requires an exploration of the nature of relationships and communication by which they seek to help others to help themselves.

This exploration is not, however, a simple journey. There are many possible conflicts between the role of the therapist, job requirements, constraints and so on, and the use of counselling approaches and skills. Therapists are not counsellors, as such, but the effectiveness of therapy clearly depends on the human relations involved, the strength of the therapist–client relationship and quality of communication. Furthermore, as Cohn (1983: 46) states: 'The way recipients (of help) would like to be treated is often the opposite of the way donors (of help) treat them.' Some of the dilemmas are immediately apparent if we consider any specific situation in which help is being given.

> Mrs Edna McBride is in her late sixties. Her husband died just over a year ago after she had cared for him through a long debilitating illness. Edna's own health has deteriorated during the last few years, particularly with the development of rheumatoid arthritis. Her son and only child, Norman, is married with three children of his own and they live just less then thirty miles away from Edna's home. Edna lives in a small council flat on the third floor of a small block of flats situated on the outskirts of a city in the north of England. Prior to his death her husband had been out of work for many years and Edna has only the basic state pension to live on. The McBrides moved into the flat less than three years ago and since then Edna has spent much of that time caring for her husband and coping with the immediate trauma of his death. She feels that she has not got beyond a nodding acquaintance with her neighbours. At the recommendation of her GP, she has been referred to the Community Care Team, for assessment in the first instance, and Ms Katie Burn has begun to visit Edna in her capacity as a part-time occupational therapist. Katie is forty and, though she is a single parent, she feels that her three children are now old enough for her to take on a full-time post. In their initial conversations, Edna talks to Katie about her loneliness and practical problems such as transport to and from the hospital.
>
> As in all such basic accounts, the seemingly simple facts belie the complexities. Even at the outset there are many diverse possibilities in the human relations of helping. First, though

we are obviously concentrating on Katie as a helper, there are a number of people who may possibly attempt to help Edna, including her son and his family, her neighbours, and also people not mentioned so far, such as members of social clubs or self-help groups of various kinds. It is also important to note that, though Edna may require help at this point in her life, she has spent many years as a helper, most obviously in caring for her husband.

Katie and Edna may not necessarily share the same view of what is or what should be happening. Their wishes, their motivations, even their fundamental world views may be poles apart. Their experiences of and feelings about the helping process are likely to be quite different as a giver and receiver of help.

1. They may differ in their feelings about how long help should be provided. Katie may be expecting to help in terms of immediate solutions to what seem to her to be obvious problems, such as practical support in getting out and about more often, and thus returning Edna to as 'normal' a life as possible as quickly as possible. For Edna, on the other hand, 'normality' may simply be inconceivable. How could her life ever be normal again? Through her eyes, she is facing a whole new life and changes in lifestyle which she may never be able to achieve.
2. Edna and Katie may also differ in their beliefs about who is to blame for any problems Edna is experiencing. Edna may blame herself for her loneliness, for instance. She may feel that she has not made the effort of making friends with her neighbours or that she has been too demanding on her son and his family. Katie, however, may blame Edna's whole situation and circumstances for her isolation.
3. People's understanding of the causes of the problem can differ in many significant ways. Edna and Katie may also differ quite radically in the extent to which they see Edna's impairment as being at the root of the problem. Katie may take a medical orientation and concentrate solely on the development of rheumatoid arthritis and all its implications for physical dysfunction. Her training and professional responsibilities, as she sees them, may lead Katie to 'medicalize' Edna's situation. Whereas for Edna herself, her medical condition may be of marginal significance to the way she is feeling about herself, her daily life and her relationships with others.

4. Finally, they may have different views about what Edna should be feeling. Katie may be wanting Edna to have positive feelings about herself and her life. For someone offering help, the whole meaning of 'being helpful' can lie in happiness and enjoyment of life for the other person. This may be central for Katie in that she sees Edna's feelings as the measure of whether she is actually being helpful. On the other hand, Edna may well feel that she has no right to happiness, that she should be depressed and that it would actually be wrong for her to have positive feelings. She may even feel guilty at the thought of enjoying herself.

Some of the issues in this whole arena of the human relations of helping are inherent in the very words used to refer to people. Throughout the book, people who give and receive help will be referred to using different terms, such as: helper/helped; giver/receiver; and, most regularly, therapist/client. All these terms carry misleading assumptions. The idea of categorizing people as 'helpers' or 'helped' is questionable. It plays a part in building stereotypes of people who are 'helped' and fosters assumptions about passivity, helplessness and dependence. There can also be assumptions about people as receivers of help, such as disabled people, which can deny that they are also providers of help. In essence, these terms can suggest a one-way relationship in which one gives and the other receives, rather than a two-way partnership.

Another major question is the use of masculine and feminine pronouns when referring to people generally. It is clumsy to always refer to both – 'he or she' – but there are also dangers in consistently referring to either therapists or clients as masculine or feminine, such as assumptions about therapy being a profession for women. In this we shall follow Carl Rogers' lead (Rogers, 1978). In the first chapter all general references to individuals will be feminine, in the second masculine, and they then alternate similarly throughout the book.

Who is this book for?

As other volumes in this series, this book is for physiotherapists, occupational therapists and speech and language therapists as well as students of these professions. The topic for this volume is equally relevant to the three professions. Indeed, it can be argued that human relations are important for all formal and informal carers and helpers. As Egan (1990) argues, helping skills are required by all professionals who try to help individuals face any kind of human problem. Professionals may be effective in the expertise, knowledge and skills of their own professions and still be deficient in terms of the human encounters involved. He lists 32 such professionals. Though this book is, in general terms, relevant to a wide audience, the particular examples and discussions are geared to therapists in health care.

What are the purposes of this book?

This study of the human relations of helping builds on the skills and understanding you, the reader, already have and aims to enable you to:

- reflect on yourself and others in human relationships
- examine ways of thinking about human relations
- explore, understand and develop your practice in interactions and relationships with clients
- explore, understand and develop your practice as a therapist in empowering clients to understand themselves better and to be more effective in defining and solving their own problems
- reflect on the development of effective human relationships and interactions within the requirements of your professional roles.

What is in this book?

There are three parts to it. In Part I, 'In Principle', we explore some of those difficult dilemmas which face therapists in beginning to consider the human relations of helping. The exploration seeks principles which respect the values, personal resources and capacity for self-determination of others. It sets the scene by introducing some basic concepts and distinctions between different types of human relationship and different ways of helping. This is also the starting point for beginning to explore your own feelings, values and beliefs which you bring to bear on your relationships with clients.

Part II, 'In Practice', examines processes of putting principles into practice. Here we look at relationships and communication which offer support and space for personal growth and self-determination. What might the principles mean in the complex and divergent world of therapy?

Finally, Part III looks at questions of putting principles into practice 'In Context', that is, the wider social context of the roles and responsibilities of therapists and the factors which influence their relationships not only with clients but also clients' relatives, colleagues and other professionals. What meaning do concepts of 'partnership' and 'empowerment' have in contexts which can be experienced by clients as disempowering? We examine the possibilities for change, particularly in the light of growing 'client power', including the Disability Movement.

Who has written this book?

There is an obvious answer, of course: I wrote it. It is not so obvious, however, when I apply the ideas explored within the book to the process of writing it, including self-awareness and communication and relationships with others. First, who am I? Mairian Corker (1994), asking the same question of herself as an author, quotes Foucault:

> Someone who is a writer is not simply doing his work in books, in what he publishes . . . his major work is, in the end, himself in the process of writing his books . . . the work includes the whole life as well as the text. The work is more than the work; the subject who is writing is part of the work. (1986: 184)

This is, to a frightening extent, true for me. This book reflects my beliefs, feelings, intuitions and understanding which have developed over many years and which I have had to confront and review in the process of writing. It is important to realize this, as the very subject matter of the book is not just academic or professional but also personal.

I have not worked alone on this project. Many people have given me invaluable help in many ways. Jade Swain read each draft and guided me from her experiences as a counsellor and therapist. Elaine Grayson, Sue Raine, Bob Fordham and Sarah Donoghue read earlier drafts and provided encouragement, examples and ideas. Carole Thirlaway collaborated with me in a research project which forms the basis for later chapters. Sally French was a great help in many ways, including providing literature, discussing ideas and editing the text, and Jo Laing gave advice which greatly improved my style of writing.

There is also, for me, a real sense of constructing this book with you, the reader. Within the limits and confines of producing and reading a text, I hoped this would be a dialogue between you and me. When I read books, I often do so with a pencil to hand to underline and react in the margin (though not library books!). You may not, of course, wish to deface this book, but there are other ways in which you might enter this 'dialogue' which are summarized below.

How to use this book

How are 'skills for practice' learnt in the arena of human relations? The book is about the skills of communication, about listening to people, and about people developing and exploring their ideas. It is also about the possibilities that exist for changing practice. It has therefore been designed as a book to be worked through as well as simply read. At various points within each chapter you will find 'Personal reflections'. These are suggestions for exercises and activities which will help you get the most out of the ideas being discussed. The approach is based on the belief and experience that there is no one, certain way of learning the skills of human relations. There are a number of processes which can be effective and which are drawn on in facilitating personal reflections.

> **Personal reflections 1**
>
> If this is to be the kind of interactive workbook envisaged, you will first of all need to equip yourself with a notebook or loose-leaf file to use as you work through. Ownership is crucial. Though you may share your notes with others, for instance if you are on a training course, the content, form and nature of the notes you make are up to you.

Developing self-awareness

This is the developing and expanding exploration of the 'self': noticing and taking account of our own feelings, understandings, behaviour, appearance, beliefs, needs and so on. Personal awareness comes both from within, as we monitor ourselves in helping relationships, and from others, as we monitor their responses and feelings about ourselves.

The practice of skills

Skills includes both our behaviour in interactions with others and the developing understanding of why we behave as we do. The practice of skills involves exploring and 'trying out' techniques in activities and role-play.

Keeping a personal journal

Keeping a journal can seem like jargon for the common activity of keeping a diary and it can indeed be similar. However, the phrase is used here to denote a more focused activity aimed towards personal development and it is certainly very different to the logging of forthcoming appointments as in many diaries kept by professionals. A journal is a written narrative, or a story, of you, your relationships and ways of helping. The aim is written self-reflection, mostly retrospective: to use writing to formulate and convey thoughts, primarily for yourself, but also for others as far as you wish or is appropriate.

A journal is a running account of 'important' events and your reflections on the events in terms of feelings, questions and thoughts about relationships and helping. The sorts of things you might include are:

- a brief summary of a meaningful incident
- important questions generated by the event
- a list of the jargon/concepts, keywords that convey the essence of the meaning of the event for you
- subjective reactions to the event
- a description of what you felt you learned.

Collaboration

We learn about relationships through and within relationships. Furthermore, reflective practice is a collaborative activity: professionals can learn more if they share their learning experiences with others. The more knowledge and experience that is pooled, the richer will be the process of learning about counselling skills. Such collaboration incorporates both one-to-one and group situations.

Collaboration requires the establishment of trust in which people can communicate openly and freely. This involves discussion and negotiation around some complex issues relating to ethics and the processes of communication. For instance, there are questions of anonymity and confidentiality to be dealt with in an agreed code of ethics which is continually reviewed. Other issues include the invasion of privacy, the right to opt out and the establishment of equity in participation so that the group or one-to-one situation is not dominated or manipulated from one side.

Personal reflections 2

If it is possible, approach someone to be your partner as you work through the text and the exercises. This may be a colleague, fellow student, client, or even someone not involved in therapy. Your partner will provide a sounding-board for you, particularly if you can work through the 'Personal Reflections' together. The partnership will also provide a focus for you when thinking about the qualities of relationships and communication. The book has been written so you can work through it on your own, but you would find discussions with a partner an effective way of taking the ideas presented here into your work and life.

Reflective Practice

Perhaps the key process in learning about counselling skills in therapy is the development of ourselves as reflective practitioners (Schön, 1983; Osterman and Kottkamp, 1993). The basic idea here is that what really matters is your development of your practice as a therapist and using reflections on the human relations of helping to aid this process. One way of looking at reflective practice starts with the idea of personal action theories. The decisions we make and the actions we take are governed by personal action theories, or our assumptions and beliefs about ourselves, other people, relationships, systems in which we work and the society in which we live. Such personal action theories include both *espoused theories*, that is, what we are able to say we believe and think, and *theories in use* or *theories in action*, that is, assumptions and beliefs which are grounded in what we actually do.

There are a number of principles behind this idea of 'reflective practice':

- we want to and can improve the effectiveness of helpful relationships
- we can take responsibility for improving effectiveness
- development requires us to enquire into our 'personal action theories' and to use direct evidence as a basis for self-reflection
- the processes of reflection are facilitated through collaboration with others.

Finally, a useful way of looking at reflection on your own practice as a therapist is to think in terms of five forms for reflection (adapted from Schön, 1983, and Reynolds and

Dimmock, 1992). They seem to summarize many of the points made so far:

1. *Discriminant reflection* is your assessment of the effects of your actions as a therapist.
2. *Role reflection* is an awareness of how you feel about how you go about your job as a therapist.
3. *Judgemental reflection* is an awareness of your own values, likes and dislikes which you bring to bear in understanding and evaluating the process of therapy.
4. *Conceptual reflection* is an awareness of the constructs which you use in understanding and evaluating yourself in your role as therapist.
5. *Theoretical reflection* is an awareness of how your own values and constructs are based upon taken for granted and culturally embedded assumptions about the nature of what we are as human beings, the nature of human relations, the processes of helping and the processes of therapy.

We shall be returning to these five forms of reflection in the final chapter to help summarize some of the main issues discussed throughout the book.

I hope, then, that you will think of this as something of a workbook and that you will make and keep notes as you progress through.

Personal reflections 3

To get into an active approach to working through this book, make a list of your own aims and expectations at this introductory point. List the strengths you think you bring to human relations, where you feel you need to develop, and also any worries you have about this as an area of study. Keep your list for reference as you progress through the book so you will be better able to track the developments and changes in your thinking.

Part One

In Principle

1

Human Relations

From a viewpoint

There are many ways of looking at therapy and all it may encompass, including the diverse range of problems that are faced, from every side, and the whole gamut of activities in which therapists engage. We are exploring one particular viewpoint: therapy as helping, and in particular the human relations of engaging in helping. From this vantage point therapy is not a set of techniques, largely medical in orientation, which can be brought to bear on a set of problems, themselves largely medical in manifestation. Rather, therapy is seen as an essentially human activity which needs to be understood in terms of the relationships, processes of communication and the people involved.

The first two chapters introduce the main concepts which provide the compass points for an exploration of the human relations of helping. Here we shall be concentrating on 'human relations'. This is a broad term which orientates us towards therapy as a social interaction involving: self-awareness and awareness of others, including experiences, actions and feelings; the personal relationships between those involved; and the two-way process of communication. In Chapter 2 we shall then begin to examine the notion of the process of therapy as helping.

Self-conceptions

> 'Who are you?' said the caterpillar. This was not an encouraging opening for a conversation. Alice replied rather shyly, 'I – I hardly know, sir, just at present – at least I knew who I *was* when I got up this morning, but I think I must have changed several times since then.' (Carroll, 1923: 73)

It was not difficult for Lewis Carroll to play with the concept of self. As soon as we begin to think about this seemingly simple, everyday concept its meaning slips away like sand through the fingers. Though it can be agreed that it is a concept and not an entity or thing, beyond such agreement lies a maze of quandaries. Alice expressed one such question: are we one or many 'selves'? I recently visited a church where I was a choirboy 40 years earlier. Was that ghost of a child I could almost see, sneaking illicit sweets and a comic under his cassock, really me? Am I the same me now as I was then? Am I the same me when I am lecturing to a group of strangers as I am when I am having a drink with a friend or at home with my children? People can seem to change, depending on time and circumstances, as conveyed by statements like, 'she's a totally different person today'.

Another question is: who knows the 'self'? Is the self what I know myself to be from the inner world or what others think I am? This becomes more complex when we take into account the idea that there are things about ourselves, such as unconscious desires and motives, of which we are not consciously aware. The Johari window activity (adapted from Luft, 1969), see below, is designed to help you think through these questions in relation to yourself. It is possible to do the activity working on your own, but the discussion you could have with a partner in doing this will be more fruitful. It is important to remember that it is not the actual windows you produce that matter: there is no such thing as a right or wrong window. It is the thinking and possibly the discussions you go through that can be useful in thinking about self-awareness.

Personal reflections 1.1

The 'Personal reflections' for this chapter are a series of experiences designed and chosen to help you develop your thinking about these key concepts of self, relationships and communication, both in exploring the concepts themselves and beginning to relate them to yourself and your work as a therapist.

There are many exercises which are designed to facilitate and develop self-awareness (see, for instance, Burnard, 1992). The Johari window was designed to help people to think about how much they disclose of themselves, with whom and in what situations. Imagine a frame which holds your world, everything there is to know about you – likes, dislikes, desires, secrets – everything:

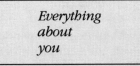

Everything
about
you

If there is *everything* about you in this space, then perhaps the first significant division is between those aspects of yourself of which you are aware and those which are not known to you. This division is clearly crucial when thinking about developing self-awareness. There is much within ourselves which we do not know, or are unconscious of, including emotions and desires. There are aspects of ourselves too which others know about us, but we do not know, including those anxieties and stresses of which we are unaware but which can easily be read by those who are closest to us. The frame can, then, be divided as follows:

Known	*Not known*
to	*to*
self	*self*

There is a second way to divide the frame. There are things that others know about you and things you keep to yourself:

Known to others
Not known to others

If we put the two together, the Johari window divides everything about you into four parts:

	Known to self	Unknown to self
Known to others	Free and open: You know and others know	Others' self: You don't know but others do
Unknown to others	Hidden self: You know but others do not	Unknown self: You don't know and others don't know

The boundaries within the Johari window can help show how you see yourself in relationships. So someone who sees herself as being an open person might draw a window like this:

Open	Others'
Hidden	Unknown

Crucial to this idea of the Johari window is that the boundaries within the window can be moved. It is possible to become more open in relationships, and of course increasingly hidden or unknown. There are two processes involved in developing self-awareness and becoming more open: self-disclosure and feedback from others.

How open are you? If possible, share this exercise with your partner, discussing your thoughts and feelings as you draw up your Johari windows working together. As an exercise it is this process of discussion which involves elements of both self-disclosure and feedback which is crucial.

1. Take a piece of paper and draw a Johari window that you feel represents the way you generally relate with others. Think about things you have no difficulty telling others, things you are open about. Think about things you do not disclose to others, things you keep hidden. Think about how you feel others might see you, in particular the extent to which you are aware of the views that others hold about you. Think about the 'others' self' area, that is, things that are known to others but not to yourself: obviously the most difficult. To get some indication of this area, think of what you might be really like beneath the face you present to others and the mask you like to see as you.

2. Next draw a window to represent you in a relationship with someone you consider close to you: a girlfriend, boyfriend, or parent say.

3. Draw a window to show how you are in a relationship with someone who knows very little of you.

4. Is there any relationship between the strength of your relationships and the amount of self-disclosure you have? How open do you think you are?

5. Why do the windows you have drawn differ? Using words which express your feelings and values, explore why some situations or relationships allow you to reveal different aspects of yourself.

Except in extreme circumstances, such as the effects of hallucinogenic drugs or psychotic illness, we all have a sense of continuity: a self which transcends place and time. What we think of and feel about ourselves is sometimes called our 'self-concept'. This is 'no more than the concept a person has of himself or herself. That concept represents how one thinks and feels about oneself – how one perceives oneself' (Ross, 1992: 2). It can be thought of as having two dimensions: self-image and self-esteem.

Self-image is basically the picture a person has of herself. One exercise which can help in thinking about your own self-image involves making a list of answers, say 10, to the question 'Who am I?'. Such lists often mention social roles and significant interests, activities and personal qualities that are significant to the person concerned. One important aspect of our image of ourselves which tends not to appear on such lists is our body-image. Perhaps the first element of a concept of the self formed by a child is an image of her body. As the child watches, feels and moves her own body, she begins to get the idea of a self which is separate from the rest of her world.

Self-esteem is the value or worth that people put upon themselves as a whole or any single aspect of their self-images. We value some aspects of ourselves more than others. For instance, I am indifferent to the fact that I cannot swim, but I feel quite negative about my lack of musical abilities. Coopersmith (1967) did some pioneering work in identifying key elements of self-esteem and the characteristics of people with high self-esteem. These characteristics are still useful in thinking about how people feel about themselves:

- a *sense of security* about self, social relationships and the environment
- a *sense of identity*, with a good knowledge of her strengths and needs, and feelings of self-worth
- a *sense of belonging*, as seen for instance in identification with people at work and home
- a *sense of purpose* and motivation to accomplish goals in life
- a *sense of personal competence* apparent in the ability to make decisions and take responsibility for them.

Equally complex questions arise in tackling ideas about what makes us who we are. What shapes the way we see ourselves? There are a number of factors which are generally held to be important in determining how we feel about ourselves in any given situation:

1. Perhaps the first are our general feelings of self-worth. These are the feelings we have about ourselves that have built up throughout our lives and are sometimes called the biographical self-concept. You can get a sense of the importance of biographical self-concept by thinking of a situation in which you have been surprised, pleasantly or unpleasantly, by how you have felt about yourself. For example, you might have experienced a situation in

which you usually feel you cannot cope and you are amazed by how secure and competent you actually felt, or vice versa. I think of myself, for instance, as someone who can take criticism. Yet I recently had an article I submitted to a journal for publication turned down with a list of what seemed to me very negative comments. Though the letter said I should re-submit, I have not been able to look at it again. I am not as resilient as I would like to have thought.

2. We see ourselves, in part, as others see us, or at least how we think they see us. A person's self-concept depends very much on how she interprets the reactions and opinions of other people, who are personally significant to her. This idea is sometimes called the 'looking glass self'.

> As we see our face, figure, and dress in the glass, and are interested in them because they are ours, and pleased or otherwise with them according as they do or do not answer to what we should like them to be; so in imagination we perceive in another's mind some thought of our appearance, manners, aims, deeds, character, friends, and so on, and are variously affected by it. (Cooley, 1902: 184)

This happens most obviously in childhood, as captured in a well-known, though rather jaundiced poem:

> They fuck you up, your mum and dad.
> They may not mean to, but they do.
> They fill you with the faults they had
> And add some extra, just for you. (Larkin, 1988: 180)

3. Other people also influence our self-esteem in less direct ways than through their responses to our activities. We judge ourselves, for instance, in relation to others, that is, we see ourselves in comparison with how we see others. If I see myself as a 'quiet' person, for instance, then 'quiet-talkative' is an important dimension for me in judging myself against others. This can be a form of 'identification'. The good feelings of others, who are significant to us and with whom we identify, are infectious. Being with people who feel good about themselves can

help us feel good about ourselves, and vice versa, of course.

4. This question of identification leads us to another factor which can be important in self-esteem: the effect of the social roles we play. Answers to the question 'Who am I?' often refer to social roles: occupational roles, marital roles and so on. The effect of occupational roles on the self-image of therapists can be seen in the way student therapists increasingly come to see themselves as therapists, or more particularly as physiotherapists, occupational therapists and so on.

5. Cooley (1902) wrote that 'self and society are twin born'. It is impossible to get a full picture of how we become ourselves without recognizing the pervasive influence of the society in which we live. There are, for instance, limits imposed on the people's choices of those with whom they communicate and form relationships. There are limits, too, on the possibility that the person will regard appraisals by others as important or significant (Hewitt, 1984). To be born black or white, male or female, rich or poor, disabled or non-disabled is to be confined to some extent within an existing network of social relationships. In particular, segregation of living arrangements, schools, work places and leisure facilities constrain or limit contact between people, identification between people, and the possible roles they may assume.

Looking at all these determinants of 'self' we can come to the view that self is socially constructed. Our views of ourselves are created, developed and changed throughout our everyday interactions with others. However, there should be no assumption that the self is without agency, that it is a passive recipient of social influences. To say that the self is socially constructed does not mean that I am solely a product of social processes. I can play an active role and make daily-life choices in these processes of construction. This belief in people's capacity for self-determination is, by definition, central to the use of counselling skills by therapists and, of course, applies to both client and therapist. The emphasis is thus on growing self-awareness. As Burnard (1990: 29) writes: To become self-aware is . . . to learn conscious use of self. We become agents; we are able to choose to act rather than feeling acted upon. . . .'

Journeys into self-awareness take many forms, sometimes triggered by traumas, and they are rarely comfortable 'sightseeing tours' and often can be expensive in psychological cost and energy. The nature of the journey can be seen as twofold and it is the interrelationship between these two which is important. The journey can be characterized as action and reflection. That is to say, self-awareness is born of the actions and reactions 'I' take and the reflections on 'me' in action:

1. The first direction emanates from the 'I', that is, the person or 'self', acting on or being acted upon by the environment, or the environment as she perceives and understands it. Self-knowledge is generated in acting on and being acted upon through experience. This can be situations in which the person comes to terms with threats and changes which are seen as being imposed. Research has shown, for instance, that severe or chronic illness can lead to greater self-awareness (Marková, 1987). People can also become more aware of themselves in the process of acting upon and attempting to 'do something' within their lives. It is through our aspirations and attempts to realize aspirations that we can realize ourselves.

2. What complicates matters even further is that there is both 'I' that acts and a 'me' that has taken the action that 'I' and others can reflect on. It is sometimes seen as the essence of being human that we have self-awareness and can reflect on ourselves. A process which can promote self-awareness is self-disclosure (Derlega et al., 1993). It draws in both the 'I' which is acting and experiencing through disclosing and the 'me' that is reflected on in disclosure. Self-disclosure is sometimes thought of as a technique used by counsellors, but it is also a process which is, to a degree, a part of all communication and relationships. It is the act of making yourself known, of being real, of revealing yourself to others. If communication is a process of sharing meaning, self-disclosure is a sharing of ourselves, and a route to self-

knowledge. Listening to yourself disclose and hearing others share their perceptions of you can be an opportunity to learn who you are. Self-disclosure also holds the risks and possible conflicts of developing self-awareness, as depicted in Figure 1.1.

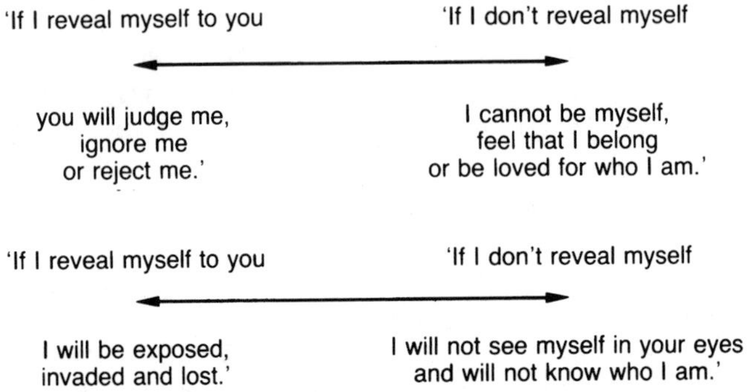

'If I reveal myself to you

you will judge me, ignore me or reject me.'

'If I don't reveal myself

I cannot be myself, feel that I belong or be loved for who I am.'

'If I reveal myself to you

I will be exposed, invaded and lost.'

'If I don't reveal myself

I will not see myself in your eyes and will not know who I am.'

Figure 1.1   *Risks and conflicts of self-disclosure*

Different relationships

Our specific focal point is, of course, therapist–client relationships. The lives of therapists and clients are, however, full of other relationships, formal and informal, intimate and superficial. Each brings to the therapist–client relationship not just their expectations of therapy but also their whole internalized personal history of relationships. One approach to looking at this suggests that we all construct a model of ourselves and our world through which we anticipate what is going to happen to us. A perspective which is pertinent at this point is Kelly's Personal Construct Theory, or as it is sometimes called the 'Man-the-Scientist' theory, which applies to everyone despite the sexist terminology. Kelly put forward the idea that theorizing is not something just scientists do: we are all, by our very nature as human beings, engaged in essentially the same processes as scientists. We are all engaged in a process of observation, interpretation, prediction and control. Each person creates a model, or 'coloured glasses', of the world in order to chart a course of behaviour in relation to it. Kelly suggests, then, that people behave like scientists and develop their own representations of the world so that they can predict and control events. A full description of the original ideas can be found in Kelly (1955) and a more recent text directed towards the implications of the theory for the practice of counselling is Fransella and Dalton (1990). Here we shall concentrate on people's coloured glasses when looking at 'different relationships'.

To prepare an example of the theory in use, I talked with Lisa, an occupational therapist, about the different relationships in her life. I listened for recurring themes in what she said about how she saw her relationships and the differences between them, noting her actual words and asking for specific examples as she contrasted and compared her relationships. Kelly's theory suggests that the models we develop are 'construct systems', composed of bipolar constructs, through which we can anticipate events. Thus when Lisa described one of her relationships as 'having a lot of warmth', this suggested that one of her bipolar constructs applying to relationships with others is 'warmth–coldness' This is one important element in the spectrum of her unique coloured glasses. From all Lisa said about relationships we drew up her grid or 'construct network'. We then used this grid to rate and compare two of Lisa's specific relationships (Figure 1.2). Relationship A is with a manager in her work situation. Relationship B is with a friend.

There are a number of points which can be made about Lisa's grid. The first is that it is Lisa's not yours or mine. You will be asked to think about your own grid in 'Personal reflections 1.2'.

Secondly, Lisa's constructs are linked together to form what Kelly calls 'networks'. The dimensions close–distant, warm–cold and easy/relaxed–difficult/awkward were consistently linked. This would suggest that how Lisa sees a relationship, e.g. 'distant', is closely related to how she feels within the relationship, e.g. 'awkward'. Thirdly, constructs are not simply verbalized thoughts. It was evident from what Lisa said that she could not always easily define or put into words the qualities of her relationships. 'There's something special about the relationship', 'There's something about her which draws me to

Close	B					A	Distant
Warm	B					A	Cold
Domineering			A	B			Submissive
Easy/ Relaxed	B				A		Difficult/Awkward
Giving				A	B		Talking
Formal		A				B	Informal
Professional	A					B	Social

Figure 1.2   *Two different relationships*

her' are expressions she used which convey the elusive nature of some relationships. Finally, Kelly's notion of the 'tight vs loose' dimension may be important in understanding Lisa's construct system. According to Kelly, a 'tight' system is highly organized and predicts that a relationship, in this example, will have certain qualities and these predictions will be difficult to change. Lisa's view of her relationships with management seemed tight, for instance, and clearly defined by roles. For Lisa there is a contrast between 'formal relationships' which are defined by 'rules and a code of behaviour to follow'; and 'informal relationships' in which 'people can be themselves'. She described 'professional relationships' as relationships in which 'people "know where they are and what is expected of them", but also as "intimidating, constraining and inhibiting"'.

The helping relationship, as other relationships, can be seen as a complex interaction between the helper and the recipient of the help. The same characteristics, phenomena and dynamics, are present as in any interaction between two parties in a relationship. This is regardless of whether the helping is undertaken by a trained professional helper, a lay helper or a friend. A relationship develops and it is the quality of this relationship which will either facilitate or hinder the helping process.

Personal reflections 1.2

One way of eliciting constructs or drawing a grid is by comparing triads of people, events or situations:

1. To explore your personal constructs of relationships first select three people that you know. You may, for instance, choose a relative, a friend and a colleague at work.
2. Now consider a way in which two of these relationships are similar and different to your relationship with the third person. Remember you are exploring your relationships with these people rather than comparing the people themselves. The quality of relationships, described by a word or a phrase, is what Kelly calls a construct.
3. Next decide what you think is the opposite of that quality and, thus, you have specified both sides of a bipolar construct.
4. Repeat steps 2 and 3 until you have drawn up a grid similar to Lisa's (Figure 1.2). You now have a version of a grid of constructs which are your coloured glasses on relationships through which you make predictions about relationships and which can be confirmed or reconstructed through experience.
5. As a final step, explore a relationship you have with a client through this grid, in the same way that Lisa looked at her relationships with two people (A and B). Put a cross along each dimension of the bipolar constructs to represent your relationship with the client. Are you able to represent your relationship with the client on this grid adequately? Are there other important constructs which come into play when you think about relationships with clients?

Styles of communication

Communication is intrinsically linked with relationships and awareness of self and others and is just as slippery and ephemeral in terms of establishing a foothold for understanding. Burgoon *et. al.* introduce their book on human communication as follows:

> Someone once insightfully said that a fish would be the last to discover the existence of water. What this person probably meant by the statement is that, because water is such a pervasive and important part of the fish's environment, its existence would not even be noticed unless it were absent. In many ways, the manner in which people perceive communication is analogous to a fish's awareness of water. Communication, like water to a fish, surrounds us. We constantly communicate with others and, except for the biological functions that sustain us, there is no activity more pervasive and critical than communication. Yet people invariably take communication for granted. (1994: 3)

In this first chapter we shall begin to navigate these waters of communication by using a particular framework which focuses on communication in constructing and defining relationships. This model suggests that there is a continuum of styles of communication with aggressiveness at one extreme, inhibition at the other, and assertiveness at the mid-point (Figure 1.3). First, we need to define the terms:

1. *Aggression* is the expression of feelings, needs and ideas at the expense of others. Aggressive communication devalues the other person, taking no account of her as a person with worthwhile ideas and feelings. It is sometimes characterized as, 'I'm OK – You're not OK' (Harris, 1973).
2. *Assertion* is the expression of feelings, needs and ideas while giving equal recognition to the other person's feelings,

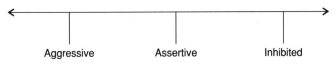

Figure 1.3   *Communication styles*

needs and ideas. Assertive communication enables 'a person to have the best chance of obtaining their desired results while retaining self-respect and respecting others' (Rees and Graham, 1991: 8). Being assertive involves the pursuit of happiness and the satisfaction of your needs, and defending your rights without abusing or dominating other people. It attempts to recognize equality in a relationship and is sometimes characterized as, 'I'm OK – You're OK'

3. *Inhibition* is more a lack of expression, that is, the bottling up of true feelings, needs and ideas. Sometimes they are expressed in such a way that they are not taken seriously by the other person. Inhibited or submissive communication can involve acquiescing to behaviours and ideas with which you disagree. It is sometimes characterized as, 'I'm not OK – You're OK', as you might have guessed.

There are problems with this framework. First, though we are looking at this as a continuum of communication styles, these terms are not used consistently. The terms aggressive, assertive and inhibited are sometimes used to refer to people ('she is an aggressive person'), sometimes to skills (e.g. courses are run in assertiveness skills training), sometimes to approaches to relationships ('she's aggressive to her workmates'), and sometimes to life positions ('she always takes an aggressive stance in any argument'). Secondly, these are not neutral or objective descriptions of communication. Aggression and inhibition can be seen as totally negative: denial of the other person or denial of self. They are, however, part and parcel of everyday communication and can even have positive connotations. Aggression, for instance, can clear the air between people. Similarly, inhibition can be valued by some people and in some cultures more than others, in that it can involve giving presidency to majority interests over individual wishes. Furthermore, aggressive communication can take many forms which might not be immediately recognized as aggressive. Aggressive communication, as defined above, does not refer simply to physical or verbal abuse. There are many ways of being aggressive in this broader sense of devaluing people, their feelings, behaviour and goals. Examples are given below, though it is crucial to remember that they depend very much on context and how they are said as well as what is said. Indeed it could be argued that communication is aggressive only when it is experienced as such by the other person or by an onlooker.

- *Being over-critical and over-controlling* – this involves communication which imposes feelings and ideas on the other person. Claims that the other person is being aggressive can, for instance, be a way of controlling.
- *Being over-supportive* – this involves communication which tells the other person that she cannot cope for herself and she needs help. It can also involve over-indulgence. I think, for instance, of the mother of a young woman with Down's syndrome who used to carry her daughter to bed every night many years after she was capable of climbing the stairs herself.
- *Being over-rational* – this involves communication which typically avoids feelings and explains away the other person's concerns. I hear myself, with embarrassment, telling my troubled daughter that she is 'too tired'.
- *Being patronising* – this involves communication which does not take the other person and her feelings, wishes and ideas seriously. Again I hear myself saying 'we'll see' to my daughter to postpone, maybe indefinitely, responding to her demands.
- *Disconfirming* – this involves denying the other person the reality of agency, indeed, of existence as a human being, and can simply involve not listening and ignoring the other person.

Communication which involves the use of counselling skills is very different from the styles of communication described above. Being aggressive, submissive and assertive in relationships is about getting what you want from relationships, whether or not you are successful in getting it. Using counselling skills is about helping the other person to get what they want and it is to this that we turn in the next chapter.

Personal reflections 1.3

1. Suggest: (a) an aggressive response; (b) an assertive response; and (c) an inhibited response to each of the following situations:
   (i) A friend promised to come to a special party, and then failed to show up. She phoned you the next day, did not mention the party and engaged you in a social conversation.
   (ii) You have bought a watch. It gains time. You read the instructions, adjust it but it still gains. You adjust it again and it stops.
2. Think of a recent encounter in which you were personally involved which was potentially, at least, a situation in which there may have been some conflict of views. Describe your behaviour in that incident. Would you describe your behaviour as aggressive, assertive or inhibited? How do you think other people involved would describe your behaviour?

2

Helping

What is helping?

Helping is not as simple a term as it might first appear. To start with, not all activities which begin with the good intention of providing help are seen by everyone involved as being helpful. Who is to say whether therapy is helpful and on what basis are the decisions of therapists made? Furthermore, helping is an activity which can take many forms and be provided in many different ways. Therapy is not a particular way of providing help but rather a range of activities which can be helpful. In this chapter we shall first explore the notion of 'helping' generally before looking at some of the fundamental issues that arise in helping through using counselling skills in therapy.

Before we begin to try to explore the meaning of this everyday word, let us listen to someone speaking from experience. This is a disabled woman addressing non-disabled women.

> . . . who hasn't had a smiling man open a door? His expectations are that you want him to, that you want his help. Who hasn't been told that women like this – women like men being nice to them, women like being told that they look nice, women don't like being dirty, taking leading roles or being without a boyfriend. . . . Do you, like men do about us, make assumptions about me? Do you assume I need help, like men assume we do?
>
> When I go out to places, the handicapist society's attentions surround me, like a sexist one used to when I was a young

girl – still does. People rush to open doors and stand there smiling at me. . . . How often have you felt like ignoring the opened door, the ladies first, the take my seat attitude? How often have you felt angry? (Hannaford in Morris, 1991: 31)

This may seem a strange opening for a discussion about the meaning of 'helping', but it is important in at least three respects. First, it puts the emphasis on the voice of people ostensibly receiving help. Secondly, it graphically conveys that helping cannot be defined simply in terms of the actions of the helper. Finally, it also raises questions about defining helping in terms of the intentions of the would-be helper. It is an old saying that 'the road to hell is paved with good intentions!'.

So what is 'helping'? How do we begin to conceive of what it involves? There are different starting points. It could be looked at in terms of types of problems such as help for financial problems, communication difficulties, problems in coping with bereavement and so on. Another possible way of categorizing help is in terms of types of solutions, including: practical help, information giving, advocacy or even referring the person to someone else better able to provide help. None of these ways of looking at helping, however, takes account of the process of change or the perceptions, experiences or feelings of those concerned. People can have quite radically different perceptions of a problem. Even people with a similar problem, ostensibly at least, will experience and be affected by the problem in quite different ways. Furthermore, the appropriate and effective way of helping will depend on the particular individual, his particular circumstances and aspirations.

Most definitions of helping seem to put the emphasis on the process of change. Murgatroyd sees helping as 'enabling people to change'. He goes on to say that 'the change may be slight – helping someone understand – or it may be a major change in the way they think and feel about something. The aim of helping is to assist people to take more control of their lives' (1985 : 5–6). Summarizing a discussion about the meaning of 'helping', MacLean and Gould (1988: 9) state: 'Helping, to be effective, has to be a purposeful and informed activity which is primarily aimed at enabling the person being helped to help himself.'

Implicit in these definitions is the belief that people have the resources and capacity within themselves to effect change: the changes come from within the client, with the helper acting as a catalyst in the process.

Another way of looking at helping includes this notion of change but puts it in a broader context of people's perceptions. Clients and helpers enter a helping relationship with their own particular set of expectations of the helping process, the role each expects the other to undertake and the outcome of the process. There will be many factors which determine and influence these expectations. The very way that the problem is conceptualized in terms of cause and responsibility will have a bearing on the helping process and the participants' roles and their perceptions of each other's role. Karuza *et al.* suggest that:

> for both the client and helper, the helping interaction is justified and shaped by answers to two basic questions: (1) Who is to blame for the problem, that is, who is responsible for the cause or origin of the problem? and (2) Who is to have control over the problem, that is who or what is responsible for the solution to the problem? They reflect a set of assumptions and expectations about the client, the helper, and in many instances human nature as well, and often imply a unique helping strategy. (1982: 108)

They go on to identify four models of helping which are based on the perceived responsibility, in the eyes of either the client or helper, of the client for the cause and solution of problems, these are summarized below with examples from the case study of Edna and Katie (see Introduction).

1. Medical model

Clients are not held responsible for either the cause of the problem or its solution. Clients see themselves, or are seen by the helper, as ill or victims of social forces which are beyond their control. Clients are seen as passive and the helper is the primary agent of change. Edna's problems, in this model, might be seen as possible deterioration in her mobility with a recommended programme of exercises or problems of depression which might be alleviated by drugs.

2. Compensatory model

Clients are not held responsible for the cause of their problem but are held responsible for finding a solution. The cause is beyond the control of the client but there is an optimistic view of the client's potential and he is seen as the agent of change. There is a belief in the inherent goodness of human nature and, given the opportunity clients will be able to overcome difficulties. In this model, Edna's problems could be seen as caused by the lack of support she had as a carer while her husband was alive and the consequent restrictions on her lifestyle. Appropriate solutions would include providing information about possible social and leisure pursuits.

3. Moral model

Clients are held responsible for both the cause of the problem and its solution. Problems are seen as being of the individual's making and it is considered their moral duty to help themselves. The client is the agent of change, as no one else should or can effect change. Edna could be held responsible for her problems as she has done nothing to improve her situation since her husband died and has even allowed the contacts with her son and his family to dwindle. Solutions could include joining a local self-help group or renewing her driver's licence, which she has not used for many years, and getting herself a small car, which would open up many other possibilities for her.

4. Enlightenment model

Clients are held responsible for their problems, but not responsible for finding a solution. Clients are held guilty for creating the problem but are seen as unable to resolve the problem and must submit to others who can put things right and enlighten the client about the true nature of his problem and the way to put it right. Edna's problem might be seen as her growing dependency on others, though no support is ready available. Possible solutions might include attendance at a Day Care Centre or even sheltered accommodation over the next few years.

This takes us to our final framework for looking at forms of helping which is depicted in Figure 2.1. This includes the notion of control of change, though it does not separate out defining the problem from defining the solution. One dimension of the diagram refers to the degree of control the client has over the helping process. At one end the client is included in decision-making and at the other excluded. The other dimension refers to the focus of helping and change. At one end are forms of help which concentrate on the problem as such, whereas at the other are forms of help which encompass growth and development for the person as a whole, more in line with the definitions of help given above. The four forms of

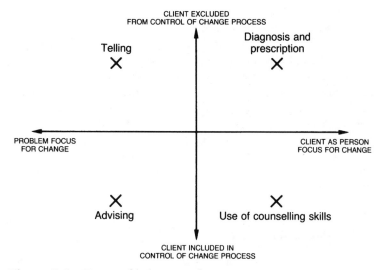

Figure 2.1 *Forms of helping in therapy*

helping shown in Figure 2.1 and outlined below are possibly the main ones therapists will be engaged in during the course of providing therapy.

1. Telling

The helper is more concerned with the problem than the particular client and excludes the client from the problem-solving process. Some forms of information-giving are examples of telling.

2. Advising

Again the helper is more concerned with the problem than the particular client, but in advising can be said to include the client in the process of change, at least to a degree. He will come up with a number of options or alternatives and make suggestions from which the client can choose.

3. Diagnosis and prescription

The helper is more concerned with the client than the problem but excludes the client from the problem-solving process. Basically the helper thinks he knows what is best for the client, diagnoses his 'needs' and prescribes some 'treatment' which involves changes for the client as a whole person, emanating into his whole lifestyle.

4. Use of counselling skills

The help is again concerned with the client as a person, but the process of help is geared towards control by the client. It is a process of helping people to understand their own motives and reasons for actions so that they can come to their own conclusions about what they will do, and how they can do it.

Personal reflections 2.1

In this exercise you are asked to review a day in terms of your experiences of helping and being helped. At the end of a workday, use Figure 2.1 and make a note of experiences of helping you have had which fit into each of the categories. Include examples of informal help as well as experiences in your role as a therapist and also include examples in which you received help as well as gave it. Then, for each example of an experience of help/helping, consider the following questions, perhaps making some notes on each:

1. How was help initiated? By whom: the helper, the person receiving help or some other person?
2. What was the reason for help being thought to be required? What was the problem? If there was not a problem as such, what was the focus of the help?
3. Who or what was to blame for the problem, that is, who or what was responsible for its cause or origin?
4. Who had control over the problem, that is, who or what was responsible for the solution of the problem?
5. Were there any differences between the expectations and assumptions of the helper and those of the person receiving help?
6. By what criteria was this an example of help, that is, how do you know that the helper was actually being helpful?

Ethical questions

At one level, the questions raised in the human relations of helping are demanding but fairly easy to identify: Am I being myself? How do I get on with this client? Am I getting the message across? Am I really listening to the client? and, as above, What types of help do I provide for the client? At a more fundamental level, however, there are complex ethical questions and dilemmas which challenge every understanding, feeling, decision and action within the whole process of therapy.

Ethics are not a predefined set of rules but rather involve continuous reflection on both the process and the results of therapy. As Churchill (1977: 873) says, it requires more than following a moral code: 'To be ethical a person must take the additional step of exercising critical, rational judgement in his decision. He must ask, "is my customary behaviour right, or good?"' This raises some of the most difficult questions a therapist can face, such as: 'Why am I doing this?' and 'What are my motives?'

Sally French (1993), in her book about practical research in the Skills for Practice series, says that the decision to do research is, in itself, an ethical issue. The same is true of the use of counselling skills in therapy, as the effectiveness of treatment procedures is usually dependent on the effectiveness of communication and the therapist–client relationship. Yet the use of counselling skills can also be regarded as unethical if it becomes a manipulation of the client by the therapist or an engineering of compliance on the part of the client by, for instance, the therapist appearing to listen to the client's point of view. Perhaps even more questionable is the possibility of what might be called 'dabbling in counselling', that is, delving into a client's personal life without his consent and against his wishes.

French (1993) highlights the following set of ethical issues or dilemmas in research: respect, informed consent, anonymity and confidentiality, privacy, safety and exploitation. These can be seen as ethical questions which apply whenever one person intervenes in the life of another and we shall look briefly at each as it pertains to human relations in helping through therapy.

Respect

Respect for each individual as a person of worth and value in his own right is a central tenet of the use of counselling skills and in general terms seems unproblematic. Dilemmas and issues become apparent, however, when the use of counselling skills is seen as part of influencing others and intervening in their lives. This is evident, for instance, when therapeutic procedures, thought by the therapist to be in the client's best interests, are actively resisted by the client, as illustrated in the following example.

> David is 14. He is multiply impaired and profoundly disabled. He seems to have no intentional communication. It was the decision of a multi-professional team with the consent of his parents, in accordance with the advice of the physiotherapist involved, that David should be provided with a walking-frame in which he should spend a period each day. Occupational therapists were consulted about the design of the frame. David, however, did not like the frame. He always cried as he was put into it and would spend his time in there making noises which would seem to indicate that he was experiencing pain. After a couple of weeks the problem had, if anything, got worse rather than improved. David would become agitated at the sight of the frame. In fact, those who know David well said that they had rarely seem such a level of response from him.

There is a real and complex dilemma here. The use of the walking-frame can be justified in terms of various ethical principles and values, such as possible greater freedom of movement for David, better access to the physical and social world and greater mobility. However, the principle of respect, or what Sim calls the 'principle of autonomy', for David would seem to imply the recognition of what he is communicating, particularly as he seems to communicate so little. As Sim (1992: 95) says: 'The right to choose for oneself implies the right to make unwise choices, and full respect for autonomy may involve allowing individuals to come to some degree of harm.' This dilemma becomes even more problematic as there is no possibility of explaining to David why he should be using the walking-frame.

One therapist expressed the issue as follows: 'It is extremely difficult to allow choices to be made when this might put the client at risk of harm.' He gave as an example the difficult decisions to be made when a client needs, according to the therapist, suctioning to remove excess secretions. This procedure can be painful, distressing and resisted by the client, yet maybe necessary for life.

Informed consent

In essence, the use of counselling skills is an opening up of two-way communication and can promote informed consent in therapy. One benefit of improved communication, as Ley (1988) suggests, is that it can result in genuinely informed consent. Again, however, the dilemmas arise when there are contradictions between, on the one hand, the use of counselling skills and, on the other, perceived professional responsibilities justified in terms of acting in the client's best interests. The latter can include 'the notion that information should be withheld from patients for fear of increasing hopelessness, anxiety and depression' (Davis and Fallowfield, 1991: 16). To what extent should a physiotherapist, for instance, spell out in detail to the parents of a 14-year-old young man with muscular dystrophy what he sees as the consequences in terms of physical deterioration if their son does not follow a programme he is recommending? If he does provide the parents with detailed information as he sees it, will this not be a form of manipulation rather than informed consent? That is to say, the parents are unlikely to withhold their consent in such circumstances, particularly if the therapist–client relationship is felt to be one of trust and respect.

Informed consent can demand an understanding of some highly complex issues. Clients who are cognitively impaired or have an impairment which affects their comprehension, such as aphasia, may never be able to give an informed consent, or the time required for communicating explanations of the pros and cons of treatment can be prohibitive. Who, however, makes the decision that informed consent is not possible and by what criteria do they make such judgements?

Furthermore, the questions of informed consent do not occur just at the outset, as may be thought. They recur throughout the whole process of therapy. It could be that the actual process of therapy is not what the client expected or to what he gave his consent. The client may, for instance, move into areas of self-exploration and self-disclosure that neither he nor the therapist had foreseen, particularly if the therapist is a good listener.

Anonymity and confidentiality

Of these, anonymity seems less problematic and does not even apply to the daily work of therapists, as they know the identity of their clients (unlike some researchers). It seems to apply only when the therapist is talking about a client with others, for instance if therapists are receiving supervision in their work. In such instances Tschudin's dictum applies: 'If you talk about your work, you should be quite sure that you do not do it in such a manner that the patient is recognised, anyhow, anywhere' (1991: 145).

Confidentiality, too, is in principle unproblematic. It is a major element in the ethical code of counselling that what a person says will not go beyond the counsellor and will not be made public in any way (British Association for Counselling, 1994). This is clearly essential to the development of trust in the relationship. Nevertheless, in practice, particularly when we are thinking of the use of counselling skills in therapy, this is not so simple, as illustrated by the following example.

A physiotherapist working in a school for physically disabled young people had formed a close relationship with a 15-year-old pupil. They had developed a high level of trust and self-disclosure, both ways, which was a regular part of their social interaction. It was not surprising that the pupil chose the physiotherapist as her confidante to reveal the news that she was pregnant. The physiotherapist felt that she had to pass on this information. For many reasons she felt that it was in the young woman's best interests to let those involved know, including her parents and, furthermore, she felt that her professional responsibilities required her to pass on the information. This incident changed the relationship between the physiotherapist and the pupil. Perhaps most significantly, the pupil never confided in the physiotherapist again and even became rather hostile to her as she felt betrayed.

In general terms, therapists work in multi-professional contexts and the principle of confidentiality can conflict with the perceived need for communication between professionals and legal and professional responsibilities. Furthermore, occupational therapy and physiotherapy departments tend to be very open plan and everyone can hear what is being said.

Privacy

The use of counselling skills in therapy is inherently a whole person approach to health care. It emphasizes the viewpoint of individuals, their quality of life, the social context and their psychological well-being. A consistent critique of health care, particularly from those on the receiving side, is the lack of such an approach. Dickson *et al.* state:

> The concept of a person rather than a patient is not fully appre-
> ciated by health care personnel and it is an issue largely
> neglected in professional training. Thus the delivery of care is
> frequently conducted at an impersonal or functional level,
> reminiscent of a production line approach, with little attention
> being devoted to the interpersonal dimensions of practice, or
> indeed to the individual's behaviour and attitudes towards
> health and illness. (1989: 6)

Yet there are ethical dilemmas here. Innumerable factors have bearing on the physical and psychological well-being of a client, including smoking, the consumption of alcohol, overwork and so on. Ethical questions come from two direc-tions: the extent to which it is part of the role of the therapist to be intervening in the whole lifestyle of a client; and the extent to which a client's human right to privacy is being invaded. Many disabled people, for instance, are very wary of a 'holistic' approach by professionals. One disabled person told me that the last thing he wanted was counselling from a therapist: 'If I want counselling I'll go to a counsellor', he said. We shall be returning to such issues later.

Safety

On the surface it would seem that safety is not an issue in the human relations of helping. This is not the administering of drugs or use of procedures which may have detrimental effects for the client. Nevertheless, there are questions of safety if the use of counselling skills is seen as part of intervening in the life of another person. There are two major issues. The first is that self-determination for the client carries both responsibilities and risks. As discussed above, the client's wishes can be seen from the therapist's viewpoint as being against his best interests. The therapist might see a client's decision not to undertake a treatment programme as being detrimental to his long-term physical well-being. The second issue is that the exploration of a client's feelings and emotions can be an 'opening up of a can of worms', that will expose problems which neither the therapist nor the client feels competent to handle.

Exploitation

This can be a painful and heart-searching set of ethical issues for a therapist to face. They range from the most blatant possibility of the sexual abuse of clients by therapists to the more subtle questions of whether the provision of therapy is more to do with the interests of therapists than clients. The use of counselling skills highlights such questions, as the prime focus is on the relationship between the therapist and the client. Such questions are exacerbated and intensified rather than eased by the notion of using counselling skills. The possibilities of exploitation are heightened when the focus is on developing relationships with such qualities as mutual trust and sensitivity. This raises perhaps the first fundamental question confronting a therapist contemplating improving the use of counselling skills in his work: What do you get from being a therapist? What are your satisfactions? This is the key to exploitation: the satisfactions, of whatever kind, of the therapist are predominant over those of the client. This is not to say that the satisfactions of the therapist are necessarily wrong, but rather that crucial and complex ethical questions are raised about who gains what from the therapeutic relationship.

Personal reflections 2.2

This exercise may help you to address those ethical heart-searching questions. In particular this is the point at which you should ask yourself about how and why you came to be a therapist. To do so, try writing a short autobiography. There are many ways to do this and it is part of the nature of this exercise that it is essentially determined and controlled by the individual. The purpose is to explore and review your motivations as a therapist, and an effective autobiography is one in which you do this. One student, for instance, began her autobiography in the third person. She felt too close to some of the events she wished to write about to write in the first person.

The following are some of the things you might do – these are, of course, only offered as guidelines:

1. First write about the key events in your life relating to your professional career. Many people find it easier to start at the present and work backwards. There are no rules about how far back you go. Certainly many of the people I have worked with have found incidents and relationships in their childhood quite significant in thinking about themselves as therapists. Some people find it useful to draw time-lines representing their lives so far and mark the key events along the length.

2. Next look for themes or patterns which seem to underpin your experiences. Who are the people who have influenced you? What factors have you repeatedly taken into account in the decisions you have made? One person found, for instance, that many of her decisions at key times in her life were to do with working and being in one-to-one situations. She would have hated, for instance, to become a teacher.

3. Now think again about the present. Having identified your themes, what do they tell you about why you became a therapist and the satisfactions you get from this work? What do they tell you about how you see yourself as a therapist and how you approach the job?

3

Perspectives on Human Relations

A matter of philosophy

Next we shall be exploring espoused theories, that is, the basic values, assumptions, beliefs and feelings that therapists bring to their work. Such sets of conscious ideas that we all carry with us inform the judgements we make in helping relationships and the meaning that experiences of helping and being helped have for us. This includes espoused theories about:

- the nature of the whole therapy process – the goals, best approaches and so on
- the nature of the systems within which therapists work – management, accountability, administration and so on
- ourselves as people and, in particular, the personal qualities that therapists bring to their work
- the nature of people – what we are as human beings
- the nature of the society in which we live and the relationship between the individual and society.

This chapter may have a feeling, then, of being about 'the whole of life as we know it' (Jim!), and in a sense, this is just what it is about. It is about worldviews or lifeviews. Peter Thomas provides a concrete example, albeit brief, of a written statement about his particular worldview as a counsellor:

My worldview is that people are basically OK, and that the world can have an effect on people that can cause contamination. I believe that if people are helped to confront that contamination they then have the freedom of choice to change, so that they can release the energy that is tied up in their defences.

I see life and therapy as a journey in which no one person has all the answers and no one theory suits all people and situations. I agree with Rogers (1980) when he says that, 'the better integrated the therapist is, the higher the degree of empathy he exhibits' and so I believe that those attempting to take others on a therapeutic journey should be travelling themselves.

My own journey is in Freudian psychotherapy and psycho-dynamic supervision. I see people as being an integration of Body, Mind, Emotions and Spirit.

My starting point on the therapeutic journey begins wherever the client is at that time. (1991: 143)

Perspectives on helpful relations are an integral part of what can be referred to as 'worldviews'. The ideas that people bring to the human relations of helping are not lodged away in a discrete parcel in the mind. Therapy cannot be detached from the therapist: her views about what therapy is, how it should be conducted and so on. This is not to say that there is always a direct association between conscious beliefs and what therapists do in practice. The links between espoused theories and theories in action are, to say the least, tenuous and complex. What we believe and what we do are certainly not always the same thing. Nevertheless, being a reflective practitioner involves exploring espoused theories, examining deep-seated beliefs and taken-for-granted assumptions. In using and developing counselling approaches and skills, we are not only meeting others we are meeting ourselves. Part of the process of learning about ourselves in helping relationships involves reflecting on and developing awareness of espoused theories. Sometimes this can be a process of clarifying beliefs which might be vague, hazy and only half-articulated. At other times, beliefs which have long been held as common sense are being challenged and re-evaluated.

A mandala for reflection

Mandala is a Hindu word which means 'magic circle' (Jung, 1964). It is an ancient religious symbol used here (Figure 3.1) to denote a wholeness not only of the self, which is often symbolized by a circle, but also of the physical and social world, also of course symbolized by a circle. The number four is significant too as it is often regarded as a magic number and again has connotations of wholeness, such as when referring to the four corners of the earth or, as by Carl Jung (1978), the four functions of consciousness, that is sensation, thinking, feeling and intuition. This particular mandala symbolizes our struggles for purpose and direction as individuals and as a society.

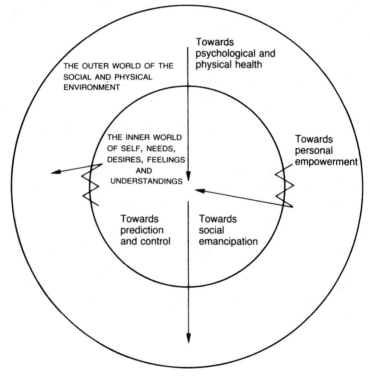

Figure 3.1   *The mandala of four directions of growth*

The mandala is offered as a tentative starting point for thinking about worldviews. It is a compass of directions for growth and change in both the inner world of the self – needs, desires, feelings and understanding – and the outer world of the social and physical environment. The four arrows show four possible directions for growth towards individual, shared or universal goals for human beings. They represent ways of looking at the world and how we see the inner in relation to the outer world. The mandala attempts to provide a compass for a self-reflective exploration.

Why, then, are references made to magic, which might seem inappropriate in a 'skills for practice' text for therapists? It is appropriate, however, given the very nature of what it purports to represent and achieve. Its substance has occupied people in thought and action throughout history, that is, the relationship between the individual and society or between the personal and the political.

The four directions can be summarized as follows:

1. *Towards prediction and control.* We strive to live in a world which we can predict and control. This goes from the most mundane activities of daily living together – to be able to drive a car, to be able to travel from one place to another – to the activities of scientists in controlling the spread of AIDS.
2. *Towards psychological and physical health.* We strive to be healthy in body, mind and spirit. Recent times, for instance, have seen the growth of keep fit and yoga clubs, and the groups of joggers on our streets. We seek to be whole as people, at one with our own sexuality and inner world of desires and emotions.
3. *Towards personal empowerment.* We strive to be part of the social world, to understand and be understood by others. At its simplest, this is the struggle towards healthy relationships and two-way communication, through which we become and are ourselves, as we are bound to and part of society.
4. *Towards social emancipation.* This is the striving to live in a society in which there is freedom, equality and justice for all. This is clearly seen in the struggles of groups, including

women, black and disabled people, against the 'man-
made' oppression they face, such as the demonstrations
by disabled people demanding accessible public transport.
It also includes the struggles of individuals against sexual,
physical and mental abuse or discrimination of any kind.

There are a few important points to make about this compass
for self-reflective exploration, starting with what it does *not* do.
First, it is not being suggested that you or your worldview can
or should be categorized or fitted under one of the four head-
ings. Categorization is for breeds of cat, not worldviews.
Returning for a moment to Peter Thomas, for instance, it
would seem that his worldview is largely directed towards
psychological and physical health. Nevertheless, there are elements which are also directed towards personal empowerment as well. Secondly, the terrain for this exploration is
fraught with hazards. There are real differences and conflicts
of belief, such as: individual interests versus community interests; and free will versus determinism, that is, the degree to
which we can determine who we are and our own lives,
versus these being determined at birth, by early experiences
or the nature of the society in which we live.

Finally, such explorations are personally demanding and
require certain attitudes, which were identified by Dewey
(1933) in relation to education, but apply equally to therapy.
Three essential attitudes are: open-mindedness, responsibility
and wholeheartedness. Dewey defined the first, open-mindedness, as follows:

> Active desire to listen to more sides than one, to give heed to
> facts from whatever source they come, to give full attention to
> alternative possibilities, to recognise the possibility of error
> even in the beliefs that are dearest to us. (1933: 29)

This willingness to reflect on ourselves and to challenge our
assumptions and prejudices is essential to learning to develop
effective human relations as a therapist. Responsibility,
according to Dewey, is the consideration of the consequences
of a projected way forward. This seems to relate directly to the
mandala as it concerns aims. Reflective therapists are not
people who are simply good at the technical side of their

work, but people who are concerned about where the whole process of therapy is going and address wider moral, ethical, social and political issues. By wholeheartedness, the third essential attitude, Dewey is referring to dedication, energy and enthusiasm. It is a genuineness in giving oneself to continuing re-evaluation and development.

In the remaining part of this chapter we shall be using the mandala compass to look at some of the formal theories of counselling.

Personal reflections 3.1

This exercise is designed to help in relating the mandala to yourself and your life. For each of the four general directions of growth, think of a specific example. You might find the following useful starting points:

1. Towards prediction and control. An obvious example for me is my continuing struggle to master the word processor and make full use of all its functions.
2. Towards personal empowerment. I think here of my mother, after the death of my father, making new friends, widows like herself, who helped give her the strength to cope with her new life.
3. Towards psychological and physical health. In terms of daily activities, I use reading and music in my struggle for psychological and even physical health with the relaxation, time and food for thought. I gain far more insights into myself from a good novel than I do from a book about psychology.
4. Towards social emancipation. Apart from people I know who campaign in different ways for equal opportunities, the person who comes to mind immediately is someone who recently left an oppressive and verbally abusive relationship with her husband after over 20 years.

Formal perspectives

The process of reflection discussed above can be facilitated by considering some formalized 'espoused theories', that is, theories of counselling which have been developed over the years in the literature. There is a whole array of theories and approaches in counselling, which may surprise someone relatively new to the field of counselling and can be threatening to the therapist wishing to find a basis for developing her practice. We are not attempting here, however, to present a comprehensive summary of the theories, but rather to help you further your reflections on your own worldviews. There is no such thing as 'the theory of counselling' which therapists can use to inform and develop themselves in their work. As Burnard states:

> No one school of psychology or theoretical approach to counselling offers *the* way of viewing the person. The approaches offer different ways of looking at the person and those ways of looking are not necessarily mutually exclusive. Which of the approaches the health professional chooses to use as a guide to understanding the process of counselling will depend on a number of factors. . . . (1989: 37)

Formal theories and approaches to counselling cannot be neatly compartmentalized. To complicate matters further, many counsellors also use more than one approach in their work (Culley, 1990). Nevertheless, it is possible to look at theories in terms of the overall direction they take in understanding the nature of human beings and the nature of helpful relationships, and also in conceiving problems and the aims of help (Table 3.1). It is to this we now turn.

In the following discussions we shall be taking each direction for growth and outline a formal theory which takes that particular track. Before we begin, however, several points need to be made:

1. Every theorist has her own ideas. It could be said that there are as many theories as there are theorists. So when we are summarizing the basic characteristics of, say, the behavioural approach we shall not be able to do justice to

Table 3.1   *Comparison of four directions of growth through relationships*

	Formal perspective	The nature of human beings	Concepts of problems	The aims of help	The nature of helpful relationships
Towards prediction and control	Behavioural	Understood in terms of observable and measurable behaviour which is controlled in a predictable way by the environment	Inappropriate behaviours learned in responding to the environment and/or lack of appropriate behaviours	Learning appropriate behaviour and/or unlearning inappropriate behaviours	Helper changing environment to change the other person's behaviour or helping the other make the change themselves
Towards psychological and physical health	Psycho-dynamic	Shaped and determined by biological needs and drives and by early childhood experiences	Repressed unconscious thoughts and feelings leading to neurosis and mental disorder	Personality reconstruction and reorientation, making unconscious conscious	Helper analyses and interprets the behaviour of the other person
Towards personal empowerment	Humanistic	Each person is an individual of dignity and worth and strives to actualize, maintain and enhance the 'self',	Incongruence between self-concept and experience and conditions of feelings of worth violated	Empowerment: self-direction and full functioning of other person	Relationship provideds a context in which the other person can feel accepted as a person of worth whose aspirations and feelings are respected
Towards social emancipation	Feminist	Values, attitudes and relationships are shaped by the organization of society and the social position of the individual	Impact of powerless social status, stereotyping and hierarchical relations including race, class, gender, sexual orientation and disability	Transforming hierarchical relationships to more egalitarian and overcoming the 'man-made' suffering and oppression of people	Relationship based on and promotes the rights and interests of both people

the range of opinions of people who espouse this approach.

2. Furthermore, we cannot do justice to every aspect of each approach. We are trying to summarize in a few paragraphs what it has taken people a lifetime's work and writing to develop. References are provided for people wishing to read about approaches in more detail. Two general texts are Dryden (1984) and McLeod (1993).

3. Overall we hope that we are providing a sort of sounding-board of ideas against which you will be able to address your own beliefs, views and feelings, and your worldview.

Towards prediction and control: behavioural approaches

This is the main direction of growth taken in many approaches to counselling, including behavioural, cognitive and some problem-solving approaches. We shall be concentrating here on behaviourist ideas and the worldview which they incorporate.

The essential starting point of a behavioural approach is what is believed to be the scientific study of people. This involves the application of techniques and principles of natural sciences in the ostensible objective study of human beings. We can understand people, and the whole social world in which we live, in the same way we understand the physical world. We go through the same process in understanding why people behave as they do as in understanding why chemicals react as they do. Behaviourism seeks to explain and predict what happens in the social world by exploring what are thought to be regularities and causal relationships between 'facts'. There are two types of facts: events or 'stimuli' external to the person, including what other people do or say; and behaviours or 'responses' of the person, that is, what the person does or says, but not what goes on inside her head. Both are by definition within this general orientation observable, measurable and can be manipulated. These facts are taken to be independent of meaning and interpretation. Behaviourism searches, as we all do, for rules which connect stimuli and responses, rules about how people learn: patterns between what people experience and how their behaviour changes. The essential rule is that behaviours, things we do and say, which are followed by desirable events or stimuli, encouragement from others and so on, are more likely to be repeated or learned.

As perhaps is already apparent, this perspective incorporates a decidedly deterministic view of human nature. Skinner states:

> The hypothesis that man is not free is essential to the application of scientific method to the study of human behaviour. The free inner man who is held responsible for his behaviour is only a prescientific substitute for the kinds of causes which are discovered in the course of scientific analysis. All these alternative causes lie *outside* the individual. (1953: 477)

Put like this, a behaviourist approach can sound alienating. We are not chemicals: we are human beings. Yet this is a process of prediction and control which is part and parcel of being human. If we could not predict and control we would be lost. If I go into a supermarket, pick up a loaf of bread and take it to the cash till, the sales person will pass it across the electric eye and I will be asked for some money. If I pay, I can walk out of the shop with my bread. Prediction and control is just part of daily living or, to extend the example, daily bread.

Providing help focuses on changing the environment, including the behaviour of the helper, to change the behaviour of the client. Behaviour is learned and can also be unlearned. Help starts with identifying the problem in terms of the behaviours of the client which are deemed to be inappropriate or dysfunctional. Changing such behaviours becomes the goal of help. This requires recognizing the stimuli which set, or lead to, and reinforce the undesired behaviours. Then, step by step, goals can be worked towards by engineering the environment, that is, changing what happens before and after actions which are to be changed. Kanfer and Goldstein (1980) and Trower *et al.* (1988) are useful further reading.

Towards psychological and physical health: psychodynamic approaches

This direction for growth through human relations is possibly the easiest for therapists to identify with, in their work at least, in that it can be characterized as medical in orientation. Growth is towards physiological and mental normality and health, though there can be disagreement over the meaning of such terms. We are concerned here with psychological or mental growth and health, but have purposely put this alongside physical growth and health, as concepts of a healthy mind are similar to concepts of a healthy body. Formal perspectives in counselling which are directed towards psychological health are grounded in beliefs about health and corollary understandings of ill-health, disturbance, mental illness and so on, and employ a medical-type vocabulary such as 'diagnosis' and 'treatment'. The most well known of the relevant formal theories is the psychodynamic, in particular, Freudian theory.

Of all the formal theories summarized here, the psychodynamic is perhaps the most difficult to convey in a couple of paragraphs. Like behaviourism, psychodynamic theory is essentially deterministic. That is to say, everything we do is caused by factors within us, such as deep-seated desires, or in our environment, such as threats, and can be accounted for. Slips of the tongue are sometimes referred to as 'Freudian slips', with the connotation that they are not accidental but signify unconscious desires. The sources of our thoughts, feelings and actions lie in hidden or unconscious drives and conflicts, often derived from very early formative childhood experiences.

There are a number of common themes within psychodynamic theory (Cooper, 1984) which help to characterize the main sort of ideas:

1. Nothing of what we do or think is accidental. Something has always caused us to act and think as we do, though we might not know the causes ourselves.
2. Everything we think and do is purposeful or goal-directed. We are always working towards satisfying basic needs and motives whether we are conscious of it or not.

3. Mostly we are not conscious of these things. Our subconscious minds mould and affect the way we perceive ourselves and others. These are thoughts of a primitive nature, shaped by impulses and feelings within the individual of which she is unaware.
4. Early childhood experience is overwhelmingly important and pre-eminent over later experience.

Help offered from a psychodynamic perspective would tend to:

• highlight the relationship between past and present life events
• acknowledge that unconscious forces are at work that affect the client's behaviour
• encourage the expression of pent-up emotion (Burnard, 1994: 35).

In the most general terms, help facilitates the development of self-awareness, the subconscious becoming conscious. Jacobs (1988) and Rowan (1983) provide good starting points for further reading.

Towards personal empowerment: humanistic approaches

A specific perspective within this general orientation is humanistic psychology, in particular the work of Carl Rogers. Humanistic psychology is a product of many individual efforts and an assimilation of many ideas. It is a multifaceted perspective on human experience which focuses on each person's uniqueness. The following are probably the main characteristics of the work of most of those who maintain a humanist perspective:

1. Attention is centred on the experiencing person and the emphasis is on meaningfulness and significance of experiences to the person.
2. The focus is given on such distinctive human qualities as choice-making, creativity, valuation and self-actualization.

3. The ultimate concern is the dignity and worth of people and an interest in the development of the potential inherent in every person. Central to this perspective is the person, as she discovers her own being and relates to other people.
4. The person has one basic tendency and striving: to actualize, maintain and enhance the 'self'.

For Rogers the essential, fundamental difference between his work and that of Skinner or Freud lies in their conception of human nature. Rogers believes first and foremost that as human beings we are free, and our freedom can transcend all those forces, from within and without, which would determine ourselves and our lives.

As in Sartre's existentialism, 'existence comes before essence' and each person is 'responsible for the self one chooses to be' (Rogers, 1983: 276). This rejection of the deterministic assumptions within behaviourism, and within psychoanalytic psychology, and the declaration that 'people are free', is right at the heart of this perspective. Furthermore, freedom as 'self-actualization' is not an underlying or implicit assumption, it is a fundamental, dynamic orientation essential to human survival and fulfilment. Rogers seeks to facilitate and empower the person 'in the direction of increasing self-government, self-regulation and autonomy, and away from heteronymous control, or control by external forces' (Rogers, 1961: 488). There is also a strong moral dimension in Rogers' beliefs about human nature in that the person is seen as basically trustworthy.

This perspective is not directed to such external, observable and measurable facts as 'stimuli' and 'behaviour'. Behaviour has meaning for the person in that it is intentional and the person is, according to Rogers (1978: 15): '. . . capable of evaluating the outer and inner situation, understanding herself in its context, making constructive choices as to the next steps in life, and acting on those choices.'

Similarly, this perspective is directed towards the meaning of 'stimuli' for the person, the immediacy of experience, and the feelings and values that pervade all experience. The person creates tentative personal truths through action and interaction with the social world. Help, then, is primarily a process of facilitating the client in defining her own problems and identifying her own solutions. For further reading, try Rogers (1980) and Mearns and Thorne (1988).

Towards social emancipation: feminist approaches

It is unusual to include this direction for growth as a goal of counselling. You will not find this in many lists or discussions of the goals of approaches to counselling. This is because most counselling focuses on the changing individual, even when change is brought about through change in the immediate environment. Thinking in the direction of social emancipation might involve changes in the individual but it ultimately focuses on changing the society in which we live.

The approach which we shall consider under this heading is feminist counselling. It has to be said at the outset, as Chaplin (1988) makes clear, that there is 'no school of feminist counselling', that is to say, there is no formal theory as such and it is questionable whether there is a recognizable unified approach. Nevertheless, there are some basic principles which we shall be summarizing, and the overall direction is towards social emancipation:

> It is training people, men as well as women, for a society that does not exist; a society in which so-called 'feminine' values and ways of thinking are valued as much as so-called 'masculine' ones. (Chaplin, 1988: 3)

Present-day feminist perspectives have emerged from collective struggles against oppressive values, expectations and 'man-made' sufferings which disempower and discriminate against women and feminist values: the struggle for equality, civil rights and 'people power'. The feminist view of the individual centres on the interconnections between the personal experiences, feelings and values and the political, that is, the social context of social hierarchies and structures. Social status and position are imposed on women, with associated stereo-typing, expectations and devaluation of the person.

Problems are thus seen as having social origins. There are social problems which are suffered in themselves: poverty, bad housing, unremitting child-care and arduous care of older people (Dominelli, 1990). Hand in hand with social problems are personal sufferings of poor emotional health, feelings of worthlessness and self-depreciation.

Growth and change is seen as being fostered in non-hier-archical and co-operative relationships in which differences are respected and, indeed, celebrated. Such relationships pro-vide a safe and supportive space for people to explore and express their feelings and thoughts and to come to their own understandings of the oppression faced through the inequal-ities and hierarchies in society. This is empowering women to contribute to the transforming of hierarchical relationships and thus the changing of society. Furthermore, personal growth and change is not seen as a linear progression, but rather a spiralling process. As Chaplin (1988: 45) comments: 'Growth is working with the rhythms, not just proceeding from some depressing reality to a perfect harmonious self in the future.' Chaplin (1988) is a good place to start for further reading and also Braude (1987).

Personal reflections 3.2

The exercises at this point are based around a series of questions. In addressing these question you might either make a few notes for yourself in your notebook, or use them as starting points for discussions with your partner. A therapist's answers to each question have been included to illustrate possible lines of thought.

1. As a therapist, what are some of your most important goals and priorities? What ideals do you work towards?

'The first thing that comes to mind is increasing the range of choices open to clients. I often see clients "stuck" with various patterns of responding which are applied inappro-priately, or driven by an inner feeling which they seek to overcome by a fixed routine of behaviours. Simply: "I don't feel good enough" exhibited by attempting to please others consistently. I don't make these conscious for patients as I hope that patterns become self-evident once the client is moving away from old patterns. This involves me in a belief that change is always possible, choices exist for people, they have resources at their disposal of which they are unconscious.'

2. What beliefs, values and assumptions about yourself, including qualities, strengths and weaknesses, do you think are most important in your work as a therapist?

'Central parts of me which are engaged in practice are a great curiosity about people. I've a sense of the richness of human experience coupled with a sense that people do not have the opportunity to tell their stories. I do need to communicate deeply with people. I feel more alive if I'm in contact with other people's stories, their deeply held beliefs . . . and express mine.'

3. What beliefs, values and assumptions about your clients do you bring to your work as a therapist?

'Therapy it seems to me needs to have a very well-defined philosophy which one needs to take on and use as the basis for practice.'

4. In terms of relationships with people, are there any differences between: (a) your espoused theory, that is worldview about people and their relationships; and (b) the expectations of you as a therapist, that is expectations from managers, colleagues, clients and yourself?

The therapist whose views have been quoted above had difficulty answering this question: 'I can relate to this more personally than as a therapist. I'm finding it difficult to relate this question to my own experience as a therapist. This made me want to go back and check I'd understood the concepts in this book!'

4

Helping Processes and Principles

Therapy and human relations of helping

Thinking about therapy in terms of the human relations of helping fundamentally challenges conceptions of what therapy is and what it does. This way of thinking is not a relatively simple matter of therapists using counselling skills to do the job they are doing more effectively. This is why the phrase 'human relations of helping' is used in preference to 'use of counselling skills'. The latter phrase has connotations of a subset of skills which can be brought to bear, like physiotherapists' skills of physical manipulations, in a predetermined process of therapy. This would reduce human relations of therapy to particular behaviours that therapists could learn, such as increased eye contact to show they are listening to the client. It is not a matter either of substituting one set of skills for another. Concern with the human relations of helping is not a different approach in the sense of suggesting, for instance, a different way of therapists doing assessments.

To conceive of therapy in terms of the human relations of helping reaches far deeper into questioning the whole nature and process of therapy. The question is not whether one particular therapeutic technique is better than another. The focus of questioning is brought to bear on the relationship and communication between the therapist and the client as people and their understanding of themselves and each other as people, that is, rather than as 'therapist' and as 'client'. There are four major elements to this.

1. The therapist is first and foremost a person. This may seem so self-evident it is not worth saying. Nevertheless, the dominant ideology in the literature, training and working context is addressed towards therapists as 'therapists', with all the expertise, responsibilities and expectations which define the role. Human relations is about *you*.
2. The same is true of the client. The therapist is not working with a disease, impairment or dysfunction, or even a 'client', but rather a person with all his values, feelings, ways of looking at the world, lifestyle and human rights.
3. Therapy is seen as a process of opening two-way communication and establishing empowering relationships between people, rather than the application of expertise by one person to determine and meet the needs of another. It is working *with* rather than *on* people through negotiation and co-operation.
4. The focus of therapy is the person rather than 'the problem': it is person-centred rather than centred on problem-solving.

Personal reflections 4.1

Schön writes:

> Practitioners do reflect *on* their knowing-in-practice. Sometimes in the relative tranquillity of a postmortem, they think back on a project they have undertaken, a situation they have lived through, and they explore the understandings they have brought to their handling of the case. (1983: 61)

What Schön calls 'reflection-in-action' is central to being a reflective practitioner and one way of retrospective reflection is writing a journal. It is a process which combines thinking and doing, or which combines helping in principle with helping in practice. You will find some guidelines for this in the Introduction.

Some practitioners, sometimes to their surprise, have found this to be a powerful process. It is to be said, however, that for those who do not develop and clarify their thinking by writing, it can be little more than a chore. The first thing to say, then, is that though it is worth persevering, if writing a journal is not a good mode of reflection for you, then simply put it aside and concentrate on other ways of reflecting, such as discussions with an empathetic but critical friend.

Furthermore, it is important not to think of keeping a journal as something which you might or might not be doing correctly. There can be no set formulas for journal writing. If it is a good mode of reflection for you, you will find your own style, content and even audience. On the last of these, for instance, one student wrote as if for another person. She addressed her journal to a pretend critical friend and found this the most effective for her. So you may find the guidelines provided in the Introduction a useful starting point, but you should develop your own approach to keeping a journal.

Therapy and the process of helping

One way of conceiving therapy is as a series of stages and as a process of moving through these stages. The usual model has four stages of problem-solving. It is a model which, taken at its most general, you are likely to be familiar with.

1. Assessment

This activity of assessment is probably the epitome of professional expertise. Though there are differences in definitions and approaches to assessment, it is generally recognized as establishing treatment priorities, sometimes referred to as 'needs', and a baseline, that is to say, a measure of functioning against which the progress and effectiveness of therapy can be measured. Thompson and Morgan (1990: 28) address the reasons for assessment with a question: 'How do we know which areas to encourage our patients to work on unless we know which areas are deficient?'.

2. Planning

Parry (1985) recognizes three elements which evolve directly from the interpretation of findings during assessment and which are commonly found in planning in therapy:

- the formulation of aims, long-term intentions or aspirations, and goals, short-term, for therapy
- the selection of means, appropriate to the individual client, by which aims and goals are to be achieved
- the devising of a detailed programme of treatment covering who is to do what, by when and how.

3. Implementation

This is obviously the stage during which the plans derived from assessments of the client by the therapist are put into operation.

4. Evaluation

This commonly involves some recording of the therapy: what treatment has been given and what has been achieved. Then judgements are made about the progress the client is making and, thus, the effectiveness of the treatment.

There are also models of the counselling process, often proposed as models of helping generally, which are likewise developed around a series of stages or phases. Perhaps the best known is that of Egan (1990). His model has ostensible parallels with the four stages of problem-solving listed above.

1. Stage one: problem clarification

This is a stage of relationship building between the client and the therapist, where the therapist helps the client to examine his views, understanding and feelings about particular experiences and situations.

2. Stage two: setting goals

During this stage the aim is to achieve a clear overview of the individual's problem, and often involves helping the client to develop views, understandings and feelings which will be useful in moving forward. It is a stage in which goals for the client are discussed, planned and set.

3. Stage three: facilitating action

During this stage the therapist facilitates the client in planning ways of achieving his goals, putting the plans into action, and evaluating the outcomes.

There are, then, some similarities between Egan's model and the problem-solving model. Stage one can be seen as a form of assessment; stage two as a planning phase; while stage three includes both the implementing of plans and evaluation. How then does a model of therapy conceived as problem-solving differ from a model of therapy conceived through human relations of helping? There are three major, closely related, differences which involve a reconception of the process of therapy when it is conceived as helping.

The first concerns the dynamics of the process as a whole. In relation to nursing, Tschudin (1991: 43) expresses this as follows: 'These theories and models (of helping) are all directed to problem *management*. The nursing process is oriented towards problem *solving*. There is a big difference.'

There are two major elements to this 'big difference' which apply as much to therapy as to nursing. The first is that therapy directed through models of helping is concerned with the person as a *whole*: it is 'holistic'. The focus of therapy is not a problem conceived in terms of a medical condition, or a lack of abilities, or a deficit, or difficulty in functioning. The focus of therapy is helping the person, beginning with the person as a person with all his feelings, aspirations, understandings and so on. Secondly, the whole process of therapy as helping questions the relations of control. It is the client's view of the problem, his goals and his actions which are predominant.

Therapy is reconceived as a process of working *with* rather than *on* the client.

Thirdly, this requires a reconception of each phase or stage of the process. Assessment, for instance, in a problem-solving model is done by the therapist to the client, using the tools of the trade, including specific tests and checklists. Part of the role of the therapist is to assess and part of the role of the client is to be assessed. When clients are involved in assessment this tends to be at the discretion of the therapist and for the therapist's purposes. The therapist remains in control of the process.

Brechin and Swain developed a different way of looking at assessment in the Shared Action Planning approach to working with people with learning difficulties. They saw it as a more mutual process:

> In general terms, assessment is something we all do to each other as a part of the two-way process of communication. We watch, discuss and negotiate with each other, forming impressions and making judgements. Assessment in this two-way sense is not just a case of you coming to understand another person. It is a sharing of ideas, in which you both gain understanding of yourselves, your circumstances, and each other. (1987: 46)

Finally, a rethinking of the relationship between the different stages of therapy is also required. As a problem-solving process, the goals and actions are supposedly determined by the assessment of the client's problems and needs as established by the therapist. This is the 'therapist-as-expert' model. When therapy is looked at in terms of the human relations of helping there is no linear model that can be followed dogmatically. Assessment is not a particular stage in decision-making but a process which is integral to the whole involvement, communication and relationship between the therapist and the client.

Structures can be useful. The models are, or at least attempt to be, clearly presented. They can help the therapist and client to move forward and evaluate what has been achieved. The danger, however, is that a structure is imposed on therapy and becomes an end in itself. Evaluations of therapy ask such questions as, 'How well have the client's needs been assessed', or 'Have the goals been clearly defined' and so on. The purpose and nature of the human relations of helping can be lost in the technicalities and techniques employed in moving therapy through each stage. This takes us back to the fundamental principles on which help is based. How is the process of therapy to be conceived and where is this process of social influence going? It is to such principles which we shall now turn.

Personal reflections 4.2

It is always useful, if possible, to apply whatever processes of helping you use in therapy to yourself. Helpers draw on their own experiences of problems, illness, stress and so on, and their own experiences of being helped and overcoming problems to aid their process of reflection. Thus you would find it useful to work through one of the models of helping and applying it to yourself. If possible this is best done in discussion with a partner who can help you through this process.

In general terms, think of an unresolved problem in your life. Apply the stages of the counselling/helping process to work yourself through:

- defining the problem
- re-evaluating the problem
- your aims and goals in solving the problem
- an assessment of the relevant opportunities and personal resources
- an action plan of what you propose to do
- how you intend to evaluate the results of your efforts.

If you are doing this with a partner, it will be important to discuss what he did to help you in exploring your problem.

Therapy and the principles of helping

The search for principles to guide the process of helping is not a new endeavour. Marsh and Fisher (1992) developed five such principles for social work practice in providing services for children and their families and elderly people. Brechin and Swain (1988) developed 'six principles of practice' for a 'working alliance' between professionals and people with learning difficulties. In both these examples the principles were offered as yardsticks against which practice could be measured. In the former the evaluation is from the professionals' viewpoint, while the latter attempts to look from the viewpoint of service users. The following set of 'principles' are offered as a basis for reflecting on therapy as a process of helping (Table 4.1).

Table 4.1   *Principles of human relations in helping*

1. To promote people's prediction and control over the decision-making processes which shape their lives
2. To facilitate people's understanding of, and control over, 'the problem', what should change and how change should be brought about
3. To promote mutual understanding
4. To facilitate people's awareness of others' preferences, wishes and needs through open two-way communication
5. To promote self-understanding through unconscious desires and needs becoming conscious
6. To facilitate self-awareness, the conscious use of self and self-monitoring
7. To promote people's struggles against repression and 'man-made' sufferings, and support the removal of barriers to equal opportunitites and full participatory citizenship for all
8. To facilitate the recognition and questioning of power relations, structures and ideologies which limit people's freedom

Principles 1 and 2

These first two principles are succinct statements of what is often referred to as 'empowerment'. This is a problematic term which we shall look at critically in later chapters. At this point we are concerned with its meaning in principle.

Principle 1 concerns a helping process which is directed towards people having greater control over and more say in the decisions about themselves and their lives. Helping is about extending choices, providing information, so people can made informed choices, and promoting the skills, capacities and confidence which people require in pursuing their aspirations, goals and interests.

Principle 2 refers to the presumptions and preconceived ideas which can determine the hierarchical nature of helpful relationships. Such preconceptions can be derived, for instance, from professional training, or from sexism, racism, ageism or disablism. If there is a problem which another person can help with, that problem must be defined by the person requiring help.

Principles 3 and 4

The third and fourth principles focus on a different form of 'empowerment'. In some forms of helping, such as counselling itself, these would be regarded as the main principles.

Principle 3 is based on the belief that the relationship can itself be a mutual process of growth.

Principle 4 gives central importance to people's aims, aspirations and goals in life as the starting points to set the course for helpfulness, rather than say professional assessments of 'need'. Mutual understanding through two-way communication again highlights the processes of the relationship itself as crucial to helping.

Principles 5 and 6

Principle 5 is based on the belief that we all have within ourselves vast resources for development and self-understanding.

Principle 6 focuses the process of helping on the tapping of these personal resources through the building of confidence, self-esteem and positive self-image.

Principles 7 and 8

The final two principles turn the whole focus of helping towards inequalities, injustice and discrimination in our society. They perhaps need more explanation than the previous principles. Focusing specifically on disability, radical changes in explaining problems, have been coming for more than the past 15 years from one direction: disabled people themselves have taken the initiative. They have done so with the support of some non-disabled people, who have facilitated the struggles of disabled people for active participation in, and control over, their own lives. Disabled people have begun to write their own history, create their own images in literature and art, and develop their own theories of 'disability' which reflect their experiences and vested interests. In doing so, they are following in the footsteps of other marginalized groups, including black people and women, as they have pursued social and political change (Swain *et al.*, 1993).

From the viewpoint of disabled people, disability is imposed on them by disabling barriers and the barriers can best be understood from the viewpoint of disabled people. Processes of changing environments through barrier removal, they argue, should be controlled by disabled people. The experiences of disabled people are of social restrictions in the world around them, not of being a person with a 'disabling condition'. This is not to deny that individuals experience disability. It is to assert that the individual's experience of disability is created in interactions with a physical and social world designed for non-disabled living.

The focus for explanations of 'the problem' becomes the barriers faced in a society geared by and for non-disabled people – barriers which exclude disabled people from full active citizenship. These barriers can permeate every aspect of the physical and social environment: attitudes, institutions, language and culture, organization and delivery of support services, and the power relations and structures which constitute society. Thus disability is created by the existing structural organization of our society and the political and economic barriers that disabled people face. These barriers are the denial of civil, social and legal rights, the denial of full citizenship and equal opportunities.

Finkelstein summarizes the development of the new model of disability as follows:

In the early 1970s the struggle for greater control over their lives provided disabled people with the experience to challenge prevailing views about disability. Not only was there agreement about the need to cultivate a new social theory of disability as a counter-balance to the existing models, but it was argued that this should guide the development of future support services which they would control. However the new model is defined, consensus is emerging that this should involve interpreting disability as the result of social and attitudinal barriers constructed by a world built for able-bodied living. This, I believe, can be called a 'social barriers' model of disability. Logically this view leads to service approaches which focus on barrier removal. (1993: 37–38)

Principles 7 and 8, then, are a commitment to a process of helping which will support people in their struggles against inequalities, injustice and discrimination.

The full set of principles outlined above is a bridge from theory to practice. They are not tied to the interests or experiences of any particular group of people, whether helpers or helped. The principles have been derived from the whole viewpoint of human relations of helping taken within this book. They point to all four direction of the mandala of human struggles (see Chapter 3). Basically, they provide a basis for action which is informed by theory.

They are, of course, very broad and they are meant to apply in all situations in which therapy is being thought of as a process of helping. This is a considerable claim! Can any list be sufficiently wide-ranging without being so generalized as to be useless? Certainly the principles in our list will not apply equally in all situations. It is fairly easy, for example, to envisage situations in which promotion of control over decision-making has a higher priority than mutual understanding. The specific aims of helping will depend on the situation and should be determined by those involved. Nevertheless, these principles are independent of particular situations in the sense that, whatever the priorities of helping, none of the principles should be contravened. Thus, even when they are not explicitly part of helping in a specific situation, it is essential that helping does not reduce people's self-awareness, mutual understanding or control of decision-making. The same is true for each of the eight principles listed: it is questionable whether any intervention which contravenes, reduces or blocks any one of the principles could be called helpful.

As you may have noticed, these principles are all mutual. They do not provide a basis for looking at helping solely from the therapist's or the client's viewpoint. The whole process, from instigation to termination, is seen as a two-way negotiation. It is a dialogue which seeks to recognize points of conflict, expectations, values and vested interests. Thus, in principle, therapy as a process of helping is not the one-way process it is often assumed to be, in which the therapist has a position of strength and capabilities and the client is dependent and weak.

This might be true in principle, but it is no easy matter to turn ideals into meaningful processes between the client and the therapist. Mutuality might be an acceptable ideal, but how far can any relationship in which one person helps another be said to be mutual? It is to such difficult questions that we shall turn in the next section of the book: 'In Practice'.

Personal reflections 4.3

1. The human relations of helping are not a matter of accepting and applying someone else's principles. This would run counter to the reflective practitioner approach adopted in this book.

Looking back at the principles outlined above, I have to ask how far they reflect my values as a white, middle-class, middle-aged, non-disabled male? Do they apply for all therapists and clients of any age, gender, ethnicity, race, culture, socioeconomic status, sexual orientation, life circumstances and basic values (Corey and Corey, 1993)? Are they in accord with your basic assumptions about helping through therapy? Do they allow processes of helping which can be appropriate to clients who come from a wide diversity of backgrounds with values which can differ radically from your own? It is important, then, for you to set out your own principles for helping through therapy. You might wish to start with the eight in Table 4.1.

- are there any you might leave out as being inapplicable to you and your work as a therapist?
- are there any you would want to reword?
- are there any statements of principle which you see as important that are not included in the eight?

You may find it useful to write out your principles in the notebook or journal you are using in conjunction with this book.

2. Given that your journal is a reflection of your experiences, thoughts and feelings in the practice of therapy, it is important to ask how these reflect your principles.

- Take each of your principles in turn and look for examples in the thoughts, questions and feelings expressed in your journal which you feel are consistent with your stated principles.
- Repeat the exercise, but this time look for anything which is inconsistent with your stated principles.

Part Two

In Practice

5

Relationships: Towards Mutuality

Empowerment?

There are numerous buzz-words in this area of human relations. 'Empowerment' is one and 'partnership' another. Even the term 'buzz-word' has become a buzz-word itself in that it is overused, ill-defined and can plaster over real conflicts and differences of opinion. In this chapter we begin our exploration of strategies for turning principles into practice and the first obstacles to negotiate are the very terms we use.

Empowerment is perhaps the most overused and problematic. The notion of empowerment is central to any struggle for mutuality in relationships, as it challenges presumptions about who makes the decisions, that is, who decides: who is involved; the goals that are being pursued; the form of help; and whether help has been effective. In principle, a shift of power is sought towards those whose lives are most directly affected by help that is provided. Given the barriers, such shifts do not come easily. It is claimed, for instance, that contracts give people needing social services greater choice, and as we have seen, choice is a word which often seems to be used in respect to empowerment. It is indeed fairly clear that people who do not have choices are powerless. Nevertheless, the increase in choices can be a limited notion of empowerment, in that the options from which a person chooses are still decided upon and offered by others. Recent research (Flynn and Common, 1992) suggests that some forms of contract do not necessarily lead to greater equality in helping relationships. Choices are assessment-led or needs-led, that is, they are still made by those assessing need and allocating resources rather than by clients.

It would seem that the principles of empowerment through help can be a screen for real conflicts, in that an increase in power for one person can mean less for another. This is in part why so-called empowerment can be a cosmetic exercise: one person in the relationship is unable or unwilling, for whatever reason, to relinquish power but still uses words like 'empowering' to describe her relationship with another person. It is for such reasons that Mike Oliver argues for a different understanding of empowerment which points in the direction of social emancipation:

> It is often assumed that empowerment is a process by which those in society who have power can dispense some of their power to those who don't have any. . . . However, it is more realistic to see empowerment as a collective process on which the powerless embark as part of their struggle to resist the oppression of others and/or to articulate their own views of the world. (1993: 24)

Yet concepts of empowerment and partnership are crucial to shifting the practice of therapy from the exercising of professional expertise to the human relations of helping. Williams conveys the 'new foundation for professional practice' as follows:

> To recognise clients' experiential knowledge as the foundation for learning, with the professional's expert knowledge at the *service* of the client. For professionals who have trained for many years to acquire a body of expert knowledge, who have passed examinations to gain qualifications and entry to the profession, to challenge the pre-eminence of their professional knowledge base constitutes a grave threat. It removes power from them and hands it over to the client; and locates their base of power with their clients rather than with their professional body. (1993: 12).

We are using the term 'mutuality' to try to express the essence of this shift in relationships. It can be expressed as in Figure 5.1. The focus is thus on the development of two-way communication and the sharing of power in therapist–

client relationships. Relationships and communication are, of course, irrevocably intertwined, but we have separated them for discussion purposes: in this chapter we concentrate on relationships and in the next, communication. In both chapters we shall be looking at the basic questions of why? how? and what?

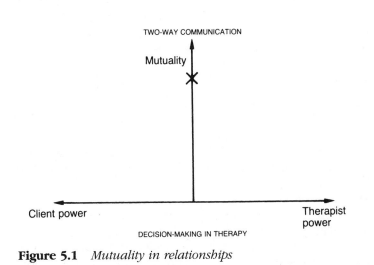

Figure 5.1   *Mutuality in relationships*

Why?: self and society

Few would deny that relationships are a source of personal growth and development, though they might equally say that they can also be personally destructive and oppressive. It is within relationships with others that we not only become ourselves but we are also bound to the social world.

Summarizing research, Argyle and Henderson (1985) concluded that if we have the right kind of relationships with others we are likely to live longer, to enjoy better physical and mental health, and to feel happier. However, it has to be remembered that these are only conclusions based on statistics. I showed these ideas to a group of students, one of whom became upset and angry. She had recently lost her husband after caring for him through a lengthy and distressing illness. This is one of the dangers of statistics. To say that good relationships are associated with better physical health seems to suggest that the opposite will also be true. Statistics may hold some truths, particularly for statisticians, but they also hold some 'damn lies' when group norms are applied to individuals.

Nevertheless, it is true that if people think of personal relationships, the list of what is gained in human relations is extensive. The question of what people get from relationships was, for instance, considered at a conference of people with learning difficulties, parents and residential workers in America (Brechin and Swain, 1987). Their list included the following.

- *Knowing who we are.* It is through relationships with others that we learn about ourselves and also, at least partly, become the people we are.
- *Affection and security.* Others give us love and emotional security, but they also give us the possibility of loving and feeling needed.
- *Sharing feelings and ideas.* We can confide in others and they in us. Close relationships can offer understanding and possibilities for talking about intimate feelings.
- *Activities and interests.* Personal relationships offer our main social activities, such as companionship, conversation, leisure, play and common interests.
- *Practical help.* Practical help refers to all kinds of material and active support people offer each other, including lending money, babysitting, pushing the car and so on.
- *Advice and information.* Other people are a main source of information and advice. People, of course, learn from each other.

Given, then, that there is such power in relationships, how are we to understand the sources of power and how it is generated between people? One way of looking at this is in terms of the fulfilment of 'needs'. We have needs which might be individual, that is, unique to a person, or universal, shared by all people, and it is within and through our relationships with others that they are fulfilled. Perhaps the most well-known theory of basic human needs was first put forward by Maslow (see Maslow, 1954, and most introductory books on psychology). He suggested that there are five needs:

- physiological needs (for food, sleep etc.)
- safety needs
- belongingness and love needs
- esteem needs
- the need for self-actualization.

These needs are in a hierarchy of prepotency. The satisfaction of unmet needs lower within the hierarchy will take precedence over higher needs. Thus, for instance, a child in school who lacks sleep and is chronically tired will not be striving to fulfil needs for esteem and self-actualization through learning. While the hierarchy of needs might be generally useful, however, there are many exceptions, such as people in constant pain who still attend to 'higher' needs.

One age-old debate which pervades the whole concept of needs is that of determinism versus free will. Are these needs to be thought of as biologically based drives which propel us along whether we are conscious of our needs or not; or are they to be thought of as goals in which we have some choice? Doyal and Gough conclude:

> What we have seen thus far is that if such needs exist, they must be shown to constitute goals which all humans have to achieve if they are to avoid serious harm. The extent to which the choices involved in such achievements are constrained by biological drives and unconscious will . . . remain an open question. (1991: 45)

What?: qualities of relationships

The question 'What?', when applied to relationships, is immediately problematic. It is a question of the qualities of relationships. We are all involved in different types of relationships and in Chapter 1 the question was raised in terms of distinguishing between relationships. Looking now specifically at the human relations of helping, how do we begin to judge whether a relationship is good or bad, effective or ineffective, open or closed, strong or weak? Such questions become of paramount importance when the relationship between the therapist and the client is seen as crucial to the process of therapy. They are not new questions, having dominated the development of the theory and practice of counselling.

Personal reflections 5.1

One of the exercises I have used to help students to think about the qualities of relationships begins with a statement (adapted from Rogers, 1961):

> If we have a certain type of relationship with the other person we can discover within ourselves the capacity to use that relationship for growth, and change and personal development will occur.

This raises the question, what is this 'certain type of relationship'? Think of a relationship you have, or have had, with another person which seems to offer you support and growth, and ask yourself: what seem to be the important things about the relationship? Make a list of some words and phrases which describe what the relationship is like.

A widely used and accepted framework for thinking about helpful relationships was first developed by Carl Rogers in the 1940s. It suggests that there are three crucial qualities which are often called the 'core conditions' of counselling: genuineness/realness; acceptance/respect/unconditional positive regard/warmth; and empathy. Rogers (1957) suggests that helping cannot be effective unless the relationship has these qualities (i.e. they are *necessary* qualities) and also that a relationship which has these qualities is all that is required (i.e. they are *sufficient*). So we should look at this way of defining the 'what' of relationships in a little more detail.

Genuineness/realness

Genuineness involves the possibility of 'being yourself' in a relationship and in communication. Genuineness in communication involves the sharing of true feelings and attitudes, or mutual self-disclosure. Genuineness in this sense implies flexibility of expectations so that neither person is 'playing a role'. When the expectations of both participants are rigidly defined, communication is not genuine. The dictum 'just be yourself' can be reassuring but also frustrating and confusing. I have had it said to me, for instance, before going into an interview for a job. It is not so simple, particularly when my preference in 'being myself' would be to avoid formal interviews. Egan (1990: 69–72) provides a list of suggestions for being genuine as a helper.

- *Do not overemphasize the helping role.* This means not hiding behind the role or facade of being 'a therapist' and avoiding stereotyped behaviours of the role.
- *Be spontaneous.* This is being free to communicate 'here and now' feelings, but it does not mean expressing, in an uncontrolled way, negative thoughts and feelings which may be tactless, disrespectful and even hurtful towards the client.
- *Avoid defensiveness.* It requires personal strength and some self-confidence to examine your own behaviour and contribution to the relationship, particularly if the client expresses negative feelings and thoughts towards you, the relationship or the process of therapy.
- *Be consistent.* This means avoiding discrepancies between your values and your behaviour and between your feelings and actions.
- *Be open.* This requires sharing yourself and your experiences. Self-disclosure is discussed in more detail later in the book.
- *Work at becoming comfortable with behaviour that helps clients.* Being a good listener does not just come naturally to many of us, for instance, and may need to be consistently worked on until you feel comfortable listening.

Though Egan's suggestions are useful, being genuine is not easy for those of us who, sometimes whether we like it or not, are in a professional role with all the responsibilities and expectations, on the part of the client and others, this can involve. The need for reflection is again underlined.

Acceptance/respect/unconditional positive regard/ warmth

This is acceptance and trust in a relationship. It involves communicating that the other person is a worthwhile, unique and capable person. Acceptance in communication also involves accepting that the other person has a point of view which, whether you agree with it or not, is valid to that person and worth listening to. Rogers himself states:

> What I am describing is a feeling which is not paternalistic, nor sentimental, nor superficially social and agreeable. It respects the other person as a separate individual and does not possess him. It is a kind of liking which has strength, and which is not demanding. We have termed it positive regard. (Rogers and Stevens, 1967: 64)

Judgement is suspended and the helper is in every way for and with the client and communicates this to the client.

A related quality of relationships is the degree of mutual warmth and satisfaction. It involves communicating the degree of commitment to the relationship and its importance to the people concerned. The communication of warmth is again not always as simple as it sounds.

1. Many people do not find it easy either to give or receive warmth, particularly perhaps within a therapist–client relationship. Two therapists who read an earlier draft of this book argued that it was unrealistic to suggest that it could be a quality of relationships with every client: 'We are paid to see these people, we do not have a choice with whom we form a relationship. Would it be expected that a relationship is formed equally with all clients? This is not always possible and could bring about feelings of guilt.' Clients, from their side, might make a similar argument of course.
2. Warmth is also felt on an individual and personal level. That is to say, there is not only the question of acceptance by the therapist, it depends on whether the client feels accepted.
3. Warmth and acceptance can conflict with genuineness. I have personally found it difficult to accept self-injurious

behaviour, for instance, such as a person who seems to be continually putting themselves down. I also have found it difficult to feel warmth for a person who is evidently abusing others.

4. Warmth and respect can be difficult when they seem not to be reciprocated. It is difficult to show warmth to someone who persistently seems cold towards you.

Empathy

Empathy is a shared understanding and sensitivity between two people. 'Putting yourself in the shoes of another' and 'seeing through the eyes of another' are ways of describing empathy. It involves both feeling and understanding how the other person feels in particular situations. It is useful to distinguish empathy from the related term sympathy, particularly when this means that one person had the same or similar experiences as the other person. Empathy involves understanding the experience through the other person's eyes, rather than understanding a similar experience through your eyes. There is what has been called an 'as if' quality to empathy, that is, feeling and understanding with the other person without ever losing the recognition that the feelings and understanding are uniquely hers and that you are a separate person in your own right with your own feelings and understandings. It is a growing together or coming together of minds, while recognizing that you remain separate. Empathy develops hand in hand with listening, which we shall look at in detail in Chapter 6.

These qualities, or core conditions, are necessary but they are not sufficient to helping through therapy. They are important qualities, but cannot be used on their own to define the relationship between the therapist and the client. They are limited. First, it has to be remembered that these core conditions were conceived and developed as a basis for client-centred counselling. Empathy, acceptance and genuineness are difficult to establish even in the specific context of counselling. They become even more problematic in the context of therapy. Therapists are, of course, not providing client-centred counselling and the relationships developed with clients are subject to and shaped by the expectations and responsibilities of providing therapy. Secondly, the core conditions do not address questions of mutuality. They are commonly couched in terms of being provided by the helper. As Crompton writes after researching the literature on empathy:

> An aspect of empathy for which I looked almost in vain is reciprocation. . . . Empathy seems still to be one way; the counsellor actively understands the client; the client's task is passive, to feel understood. (1992: 32)

It is the helper who provides the empathy, acceptance and genuineness. This can be one-sided. Helping relations are, in principle, mutual and mutuality requires a two-way flow of warmth, empathy, respect and genuineness.

Personal reflections 5.2

The application of principles into practice is problematic. There are real conflicts and dilemmas: dilemmas for you when there are inconsistencies in your feelings, beliefs and understandings about yourself, the client and the process of therapy; conflicts or differences between your feelings, beliefs and understandings and those of the client; and difficulties when account has to be taken of the views of others involved, members of the family or other professionals for instance.

The following activity can be undertaken alone, but could also form the basis for discussions with your partner.

1. Select one of the core conditions.
2. Think of a relationship, preferably as part of your work, with a colleague, parent or client, in which you have found it difficult to establish the core conditions, that is the relationship lacks empathy, warmth and acceptance, or genuineness.
3. How do you feel about the other person? Where do you think the problem lies? How do you behave towards the other person?

4. Now answer the same questions trying to take the other person's point of view: how does the other person feel about you?, etc.
5. It can help to compare relationships. Think of a second relationship, but this time one which does have this quality or core condition. How are the two relationships similar and how do they differ? How do you differ in the two relationships?

How?: a working alliance

The term 'working alliance', borrowed from a paper by Brechin and Swain (1988), is used here to characterize a relationship based on mutuality. However, as we have been arguing, to suggest that relationships between therapists and clients are 'mutual' is deeply problematic and can maintain the status quo and even strengthen inequalities. To declare a relationship to be equal, in which all decisions are negotiated and agreed, can suppress criticism and conflict. People cannot easily question that which they have ostensibly agreed to. For me, one of the motivations for writing this book is to counteract the idea that using counselling skills is a matter of therapists simply drawing on skills and techniques which further the work they are already doing with clients. To look at therapy in the light of human relations of helping is to challenge assumptions about the whole nature and process of therapy.

The barriers to mutuality are constructed in numerous beliefs and assumptions:

- the client has physical and psychological 'problems': the therapist is well adjusted physically and psychologically
- the client needs help: the therapist can provide help
- the client is dependent: the therapist has power
- the client is an individual: the therapist can call upon colleagues and other professionals
- the client only has her own experiences and feelings: the therapist has a body of knowledge and research about therapy

- the client can be physically vulnerable, being in need of intimate bodily care: the therapist is physically in control of procedures which can involve intimate contact with the client
- the client is psychologically vulnerable and experiencing any number of emotions including anxiety, fear and guilt: the therapist is psychologically in control and has little emotional interest in the relationship
- the client is experiencing a whole turning point of readjustment in life in which dearly held values and beliefs are being challenged: the therapist is doing her job.

In such contexts, a working alliance between therapist and client is an ideal. The elements or ingredients of such a relationship have been discussed by, among others, Davis (1993). In his 'partnership model', he includes: working closely, common aims, complementary expertise, mutual respect, negotiation, communication, honesty and flexibility. He suggests that what is required is 'an explicit understanding of the nature of the relationship for which we strive' (1993: 37). The actual term 'working alliance' has been quite widely used and developed in the literature. Woody *et al.* (1989), who trace its origins to psychodynamic theory, discuss three aspects of the alliance with respect specifically to counselling: agreement over mutual goals; mutual understanding of the tasks of each person; and the bonds of liking, caring and trusting that the counsellor and client share.

There are, then, ideas which can be drawn on in understanding what a 'working alliance' involves. However, any such understanding has to be tentative and the subject of continuous reflection rather than being a set of pre-established rules about how relationships should be established. There is no such thing as 'the effective relationship'. Each relationship is constructed afresh between the therapist and the client and all that can be offered is a tentative model for striving towards a working alliance.

A tentative model

A tentative model of a working alliance is summarized in Table 5.1. As you will immediately see, it is based on the 'principles of helping' which were laid out in Chapter 4. The helping relationship needs first of all to be based within principles of what is being striven for in helping. It is here that a working alliance is meaningful rather than being an end in its own right. A different set of principles would require different relationships. An expert model of therapy, for instance, would require a more autocratic, hierarchical type of relationship.

We shall look then in a little more detail at the relationship described in each part of the table.

1. The relationship provides a basis for the enhancement of decision-making control by people over their own lives
2. The relationship facilitates in defining the goals of help, and deciding how they are to be achieved and whether they have been achieved.

A working alliance must in the first instance be founded on a negotiation of what the process of helping is working towards. Without this, preconceptions and expectations from both sides can pull in opposite directions. Uneasy alliances are built on conflicting preconceptions of the problem, possible solutions and the control of the process. The principles of helping do not require the therapist and client to have common goals but rather an open two-way flow of communication in which each is able and enabled to explore their perceptions of the problem, the goals of helping and the decision-making process.

3. The relationship provides a context in which both feel accepted as a person of worth and value whose aspirations, capabilities and feelings are respected, and is based on mutual warmth and satisfaction.
4. The relationship is one in which both can 'be themselves' and be genuine in sharing true feelings and attitudes.
5. The relationship is built on and promotes shared understanding and mutual sensitivity between both people.

Table 5.1 *A tentative model of a working alliance*

Principles of helping	Processes/qualities of helpful relationships
1. To promote people's prediction and control over the decision-making processes which shape their lives	The relationship provides a basis for the enhancement of decision-making control by people over their own lives
2. To facilitate people's understanding of, and control over, 'the problem', what should change and how change should be brought about	The relationship facilitates in defining the goals of help, and deciding how they are to be achieved and whether they have been achieved
3. To promote mutual understanding	The relationship provides a context in which both feel accepted as a person of worth and value whose aspirations, capabilities and feelings are respected
4. To facilitate people's awareness of others' preferences, wishes and needs through open two-way communication	The relationship is one in which both can be themselves and be genuine in sharing true feelings and attitudes
	The relationship is built on and promotes shared understanding and mutual sensitivity between both people
	The relationship is based on and provides a degree of mutual warmth and satisfaction
5. To promote self-understanding through unconscious desires and needs becoming conscious	The relationship provides a context in which self-awareness is enhanced through awareness of the other person and awareness of the relationship itself
6. To facilitate self-awareness, the conscious use of self and self-monitoring	The relationship itself enhances self-esteem
7. To facilitate the recognition and questioning of power relations, structures and ideologies which limit people's freedom	The relationship itself is based on a recognition of the rights, responsibilities and interests of both people
8. To promote people's struggles against repression and 'man-made' sufferings, and support the removal of barriers to equal opportunities and full participatory citizenship for all	The relationship provides a context in which the constraints and barriers facing both people can be openly discusssed and questioned
	The relationship provides processes of support in promoting the rights and interests of both people

These elements of a working alliance are based on the three core conditions of relationships discussed above. When people think about mutual relationships, as in 'Personal reflection 5.1', two qualities of relationships are repeatedly mentioned: trust and sensitivity. Neither is easily established of course. Bennett (1993: 36) provides a typical list of strategies for encouraging trust:

- being sensitive to the person's needs and feelings
- demonstrating genuineness and sincerity
- being realistic, but optimistic, about people's abilities to get to grips with the problems they face
- maintaining confidentiality
- making a contract and keeping any agreements made.

Ways for encouraging sensitivity must first of all involve being with the other person: shared activities and shared experience. There are many possibilities, depending on individuals and circumstances. Dalton (1994: 119) has definite preferences: 'The most powerful medium of all for sharing is music. Listening to music together can form a bond of feeling and understanding like nothing else for some.'

Brechin and Swain (1987: 47) suggest that such sharing is part of getting to know each other which allows you to see:

- what someone notices or reacts to
- what they seem to like or not like
- what they try to do
- what they manage to do
- what they seem to understand
- how they show their reactions and feelings
- how they react to you in different situations.

Though these and other strategies may be useful, trust and sensitivity depend, in the first instance, on the establishment of a two-way flow of communication (the specific focus for the next chapter).

6. The relationship provides a context in which self-awareness is enhanced through awareness of the other person and awareness of the relationship itself.
7. The relationship itself enhances self-esteem.

The focus here is on reflection and facilitating reflection. With a working alliance as an ideal, therapists need to look at themselves, their beliefs, their feelings and their actions. Again, given that the whole context of therapy puts the power and control in the hands of therapists, any move towards a working alliance requires them to reflect on themselves as people and their practice as therapists.

8. The relationship itself is based on a recognition of the rights, responsibilities and interests of both people.
9. The relationship provides a context in which the constraints and barriers facing both people can be openly discussed and questioned.
10. The relationship provides processes of support in promoting the rights and interests of both people.

Many different kinds of feminist activism have incorporated such principles and questioned all forms of hierarchy in interpersonal relationships. For instance, the following is a list of strategies for establishing egalitarian processes in women's groups which would seem to apply to the forming and maintenance of any mutual relationship (Dominelli, 1990: 83):

• sensitivity to privileges, differential access to resources, and other forms of inequality between women and seeking ways of overcoming them
• sensitivity to differences between women, especially those based on social divisions such as class, 'race', age and sexual orientation
• sensitivity to other women's difficulties in expressing themselves and support in overcoming them
• developing individual women's strength and confidence
• sharing skills and knowledge
• open discussions
• not blaming women for their oppression.

Looking at this 'tentative model' we need to ask: do these 10 statements describe a mutual relationship in all circumstances? The answer is 'tentatively', in that there can be no definitive set of statements which can take account of every situation that you might encounter as a therapist. The model can only be an aid in the processes of reflection and developing self-awareness that therapists engage in. It is a set of statements which are founded on values that you or your clients may not share, coming perhaps from very different cultural backgrounds. Corey and Corey (1993) provide examples of assumptions which may interfere with helping in multi-cultural situations, including the following.

1. Assumptions about trusting relationships

As a helper you may form relationships quickly and expect yourself and your clients to talk easily about your personal lives. This may be difficult for some clients who expect meaningful relationships to be slow to form and for clients from cultures in which trust is to be earned rather than assumed.

2. Self-actualization

The belief in the importance of the individual is not shared equally across all cultures. Clients may be more concerned about how changes might affect others in their lives. Value systems can differ quite fundamentally in terms of whether self-worth is an individual or a collective matter and whether the greatest priority is given to the betterment of the group or of the individual.

3. Assumptions about directness

Corey and Corey state:

> Although the Western orientation prizes directness, some cultures see it as a sign of rudeness and as something to be avoided. If you are not aware of this cultural difference, you could make the mistake of interpreting a lack of directness as a sign of being unassertive, rather than as a sign of respect. (1993: 117)

4. Assumptions about assertiveness

The ideal of determining your life and telling others what you think and feel is not shared across all cultures.

In a reflective practitioner approach a key to striving against unintentional racism, disablism, sexism and ageism lies in challenging basic underlying assumptions, often accepted as common sense. The purpose of the tentative model is to facilitate this reflective process.

Personal reflections 5.3

In your journal writing concentrate for a while on your relationships with clients. Think about the following questions in relation to each event you record:

1. What evidence is there of the three core conditions in your relationship with the client?
2. What evidence is there that you (and the client) have had difficulties in establishing the core conditions?
3. What are your feelings in terms of the sufficiency of the core conditions. Look through the full list of processes/qualities of helpful relationships (Table 5.1) and make a note of any of the others which are already important, or should be made more important, in this particular relationship.
4. Is there anything about this particular relationship which has implications for how you think about and act in other relationships?
5. Is there anything about other relationships you have which is useful in understanding the qualities and processes of this particular relationship?

6

Communication: Towards Two-way Flow

What is 'communication'?

The complexities of interpersonal communication, that is not including the media, are such that it defies clear definition. It is elusive because it happens *between* people. It cannot be defined simply by the behaviour of an individual. A smile might be an act of communication, but depending on the context, the same act can convey anything from affection, to threat, to lack of understanding, to embarrassment, as well as mixed messages. Nor can it be defined by the intentions of the individuals involved. A look on someone's face, a touch or a wave of the hand can convey a whole array of messages about feelings and attitudes of which the sender is unaware. It cannot be defined either by the form that messages take. Everything about people and everything they do, from the style of their hair, to their accents, to the way they stand can convey messages. We have to complicate this seemingly endless list even further by adding written communication, drama, music, and the ever expanding technology of communication through faxes, computers and so on. A few lines of poetry, for instance, can touch on feelings and shared understandings which an hour of conversation might never reach.

The complications of communication become even more ravelled when it is placed within the whole umbrella of human relations. Marková writes:

Interpersonal communication is one of the most significant expressions of self- and other-awareness. Its quality and kind depend very largely on the participants' ability to assess each other's feelings, thoughts and intentions, and on their reactions to each other's messages. (1987: 134)

Communication is closely related to concept of self, self-awareness and awareness of others. This has three elements:

1. The messages we intentionally attempt to convey are shaped by self-awareness of thoughts, feelings and sensations. For instance, to convey intentionally the message that you are feeling anxious about a certain situation relies, in the first instance, on you being aware of feelings of anxiety.
2. The act of communication can in itself increase self-awareness. Thus, for instance, I might not know how I feel about a certain situation until I have talked it over with a confidante.
3. Furthermore, our conceptions of ourselves, self-image and self-esteem, are at least in part determined by the responses of others (see Chapter 1).

Communication also has meaning in the context of relationships. This is easy to see: you need only compare one of those long difficult conversations in which you remain 'in the dark' with a 'look in the eyes' of an intimate partner which conveys a whole world of meaning. The following extract from Tolstoy's *Anna Karenin* uses a compelling example of communication in a close relationship:

'Here,' he said, and wrote down the initial letters, w,y,t,m,i,c,n,b – d, t, m, n, o, t? These letters stood for, 'When you told me *it could not be* – did that mean never or then?' There seemed no likelihood that she would be able to decipher this complicated sentence; but he looked at her as though his life depended on her understanding the words.

She gazed up at him seriously, then leaned her puckered forehead on her hand and began to read. Once or twice she stole a look at him, as though asking, 'Is it what I think?'

'I know what it is,' she said flushing a little.

'What is this word?' he said, pointing to the n which stood for *never*.

'That means *never*,' she said, 'but it's not true!' (Tolstoy, 1954: 422–423)

Speech and language therapists could also give many examples of children whose speech is incomprehensible to strangers and yet they are easily understood by people close to them, such as their parents.

Finally, in this list of complexities, wider issues must come into play. Communication is defined by the whole social and historical context. It is culturally defined: a way of dressing or a hand gesture, for instance, can have quite different connotations in one culture than in another.

This discussion of the definition of 'communication' is not an academic exercise to attempt to produce a definitive version. It has real implications for the pursuit of effective human relations of helping in therapy. If communication is defined in terms of conveying messages, the implication is that effective communication is dependent on the skills of the therapist and the client in conveying and understanding messages. This is, however, too simplistic. The complex, delicate and subtle processes of communication can be distorted and blocked in many ways:

- the client's difficulties in expression, including a whole range of impairments from stuttering, to lack of speech, to lack of control over movements of the body and so on
- the client's difficulties in comprehension, including learning difficulties, hearing impairment, visual impairment and so on
- the therapist's difficulties in expression, including use of jargon, patriarchical attitudes and so on
- the therapist's difficulties in comprehension, including lack of time to listen, preconceptions and so on.

Such problems can, of course, be the main focus for therapy itself, particularly for speech and language therapists. We are not attempting, however, to provide a comprehensive discussion of all such problems. This would go well beyond the scope and orientation of the book. Focusing on two-way communication as part of the human relations of helping, we are concentrating on the processes of communication themselves. This is not to deny that there are 'problems' as listed above, but rather to return to the assertion that communication happens *between* people and these problems need to be understood in this wider context. The crucial questions in improving the effectiveness of communication are about the general processes: the questions of why we communicate, what is communicated and how we communicate, and it is to these that we shall now turn.

Why?: constructing relationships

Why do we communicate? The question is so basic that it defies answers. As Dalton (1994: 1) says: 'Spoken and written language are the media through which we learn to co-operate with one another and organise ourselves socially.' Yet the question of why is crucial in that the purposes of communication determine both what is communicated and how it is communicated. Perhaps the most fundamental barrier to communication is the lack of a reason to communicate.

Purpose in communication can be looked at in terms of what a person consciously wishes to communicate to another. There are times when it seems useful to consider what we intend to communicate, for example when preparing a report. Indeed, intentional communication tends to be given priority in training and literature aimed at professionals and managers. Torrington (1982), for instance, argues that the most important issue for a person in charge is to have a clear understanding of his role in any interaction with others. Each possible role can be associated with a style of interaction as follows:

Role of principal	*Type of interaction*
Tutor	Training for skill
Exponent	Making a speech
Selector	The selection interview
Investigator	The attitude survey
Counsellor	Counselling
Monitor	Discipline
Negotiator	Negotiation
Arbitrator	Arbitration

This type of breakdown can be useful in considering intentional communication. It is of limited value, as so much communication is unintentional, and indeed it can be quite difficult to distinguish between the intended and unintended in the flow of face-to-face communication. If you think that everything we are and do can communicate – clothes, posture, tone of voice, facial expression, eye contact and so on – it soon becomes evident that distinguishing between intentional and unintentional communication is no simple matter. How much of what we communicate by the way we dress, for instance, is intended and how much is unintended?

Another way of looking at the purposes of communication is in terms of functions, intended or not, that communication serves. This has received much attention. Searle (1976), for instance, suggests five types of use to which language is put:

- *representatives* – an assertion; a belief that something is true
- *directives* – an order or command made to the listener; may also be requests and questions
- *commissions* – commitments to be fulfilled in the future; vows, promises
- *expressives* – statements of feeling about an event; apologies, statements of apprehension
- *declarations* – words that bring change or a new state of affairs; judges' rulings, church edicts and so on.

Penman (1980) makes a useful distinction between functions associated with the activity/concerns of the participants (activity-orientated) and functions associated with the relationship between the participants (relation-orientated). Both functions are served at the same time in any process of communication. He suggests three activity-orientated functions:

- the task to be accomplished
- the problems/concerns of the participants
- the expansion of available alternative solutions.

He also identifies three relation-orientated functions:

- defining
- maintaining
- or redefining the social relationship.

Watzlawick *et.al.* provide an example:

> If woman A points to woman B's necklace and asks, 'Are those real pearls?', the content of her question is a request for information about an object. But at the same time she also gives – indeed cannot **not** give – her definition of the relationship. How she asks (especially, in this case, the tone and stress of voice, facial expression, and context) would indicate comfortable friendliness, comparativeness, formal business relations, etc. (1967: 84)

In this example, the activity-oriented function is 'the problems/concerns of the participants', specifically the nature of woman B's necklace. The relation-oriented function will obviously depend on their existing relationship, as to whether it is being defined, maintained or redefined. As this example also illustrates, the relation-oriented functions tend to be nonverbal and depend on how we communicate or on communication styles.

In therapy, too, whatever the activity-orientated function of communication, such as assessment, planning or evaluation, there is always a relation-oriented function. The relationship between the therapist and the client is defined or maintained through all the communication between them.

What?: meanings and feelings

Communication is sometimes thought of as the sending and receiving of messages between people, but this does not fully reflect the processes of communication and can be misleading if it is taken too literally. Sending and receiving a message can be thought of as like the sending and receiving of a parcel. However, if I communicate a message to you I still have that message. To communicate is to share – to share thoughts, feelings, information and so on. Indeed when two people communicate very effectively they are sometimes said to 'be of a like mind'.

Communication, then, takes place in a context which gives meaning to 'messages', and meanings are constructed and shared between people. With most people with whom we communicate there is an overlap. We share the same language, understand the same social rules, and have some common experiences of family, school and so on.

Looking specifically at non-verbal communication, there are a number of answers to the question 'What?' First, non-verbal behaviours accompany, elaborate on and manage speech. For instance, Ekman and Friesen (in Hall and Hall, 1988) distinguish between three types of hand gestures:

- those which can be directly translated into words or phrases, such as 'hello', 'stop' or some ruder examples which are well known
- those which add directly to the meaning of speech, e.g. by adding emphasis or pointing out directions being given verbally
- those which are self-orientated, such as stroking your hair, pulling your ear or scratching.

Non-verbal communication also manages the flow of communication. Eye contact, for instance, is involved in managing turn-taking, that is, signalling when one person is to stop speaking and the other to start. Non-verbal behaviours also accompany speech by sending feedback signals of boredom, incredulity, joy and so on.

Non-verbal behaviours play a key role in expressing both interpersonal attitudes and emotions. In relation to the former, Trower *et al.* (1978: 16), summarizing research at that time, suggested that there are two dimensions of attitudes, as shown in Figure 6.1. Attitudes of superiority/dominance can be expressed, for instance, through invasion of the other person's personal space or staring. Liking/warmth can be expressed in eye contact, touch, facial expression and so on. Emotional states, such as anger, depression, anxiety, joy and fear, can also find a communication outlet through non-verbal channels, whether or not the communication is purposeful. Anger, for instance, can be conveyed through no more than a flash of the eyes.

Two crucial points emerge at this stage. First, there is no simple one-to-one correspondence between non-verbal behaviours and the meaning expressed. The context is all-important. Even signals which usually have a well-defined

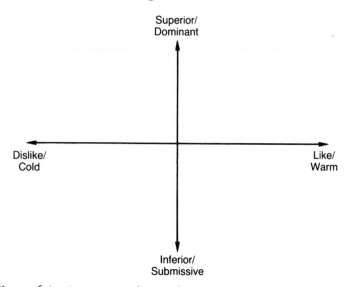

Figure 6.1 *Interpersonal attitudes*

meaning, such as raising the hand to signal 'stop', depends on the context of the whole two-way flow; for instance, if accompanied by a smile the raising of the hand could be taken as a joke. Furthermore, there are real differences between cultures in the actual behaviours used and their possible meanings. Unlike British children, for instance, black Americans, Puerto Ricans and Japanese children tend to avert their eyes when listening to another person. This can be understood by British adults to be a sign that the child is not listening or, even worse, is purposefully showing that he is not listening. Similarly, white English and Americans require a much larger personal space and they also touch less than people from some other cultures. Thus, there is plenty of room for misunderstanding and the need for reflection and feedback to check understanding is essential.

Secondly, it is also clear that there are numerous points in therapist–client interactions at which non-verbal behaviours, through intent or otherwise, can convey a hierarchical, de-personalized relationship. Clients' dependence, powerlessness and inferiority can be expressed and constructed through professional uniforms and equipment, proximity, touch and so on.

How?: by all means

Communication is such an important part of our existence that it is difficult, if not impossible, to say when a person is not communicating. If we were to meet, rather than communicate through this text, everything about me would be sending messages to you even before I opened my mouth to speak. But what was communicated would depend on you as well as me. What was communicated would be shaped by your previous experiences and expectations and your interpretation of what I do and how I look. It would also depend on my responses to you, or your interpretations of my responses. It is not surprising, then, that we are often unaware of how much we communicate to each other.

There are numerous channels of interpersonal communication. The most obvious is verbal communication: what is expressed in the meaning of words. Important as this is, however, many people who investigate communication come to believe that the most important channels for conveying meaning are non-verbal. One way of categorizing all the different types of non-verbal behaviour is in three groups (Figure 6.2) (Trower *et al.*, 1978).

The first category is called 'vocal', though it is often referred to as 'paralanguage'. This covers all those aspects of speech and the sounds we make which convey meaning other than the words actually spoken: 'It's not what you say, it's the way that you say it.' This includes: loudness, pitch, intonation, emotional quality, stress and accent.

Stress, for instance, can alter the meaning of a statement quite considerably. Take the sentence, 'I gave John the pen'. Say this statement with a strong stress on the word 'I' and you convey that it was 'I' and not somebody else who gave John the pen. Put the stress on 'gave' and the meaning now changes to emphasizing that the pen was given rather than, say, sold or lent. Put the stress on 'John' and it means that it was he as

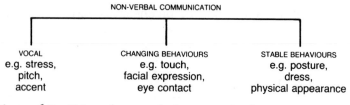

Figure 6.2   *Types of non-verbal communication*

opposed to somebody else to whom the pen was given. Finally, put the stress on 'the pen' and this conveys that it was a pen rather than a pencil or anything else that had been given. Similarly, the statement can be said loudly and angrily and mean, perhaps, that he had no right to lose it as it had been given to him. Again the statement might be said in such a way, particularly with accompanying facial expression, that conveys that the speaker is lying: he did not give John the pen at all. This is sometimes called 'leakage', that is, when non-verbal behaviour sends messages without the speaker knowing.

The second category of non-verbal behaviours, 'changing behaviours', tends to be the best known and talked about. Eyes, for instance, have been called the window to the soul, and eye contact is an extremely expressive means of non-verbal communication. All the emotions, including affection, anger, fear and joy, can be there in the eyes. Facial expression is also a powerful channel with, generally, a tremendous range of expressions for conveying messages, responses, attitudes and emotions.

One particularly complex channel of communication for therapists is touch. It is another potentially very powerful channel: a single touch can say more than a thousand words. It can also be a major part of the therapist's work. The situation is made even more complex by the sexual implications and taboos of some forms of touch. Proximity is also important in this context. MacWhannell (1192: 103) writes: 'Physiotherapists have the privilege of intruding upon the customary space people maintain around themselves, that is their "personal space".' Being repeatedly subjected to impersonal touch and being intruded upon can have implications for how clients feel about themselves and their bodies.

The third category of non-verbal behaviours includes those which generally remain the same throughout a period of inter-action, including: dress, posture, hairstyle and so on. French (1992) has written on the subject of dress, particularly uni-forms, and what she calls, 'professional trappings' such as para medical equipment and badges. Such non-verbal mes-sages can, she suggests, help to create a hierarchical relation-ship and psychological distance between therapist and client.

Opening channels

Our explorations of the ways in which the channels of inter-personal communication can be opened up began in the pre-vious chapter. Relationships are not only defined and maintained through communication, but communication is constructed within relationships. Trust in a relationship, for instance, is built up through communication, at least in part, but also trust in a relationship is a foundation stone for com-munication. Such is the reciprocal interplay of relationships and communication. Opening a two-way flow of communica-tion goes hand in hand with the establishment of a mutual relationship, as described in the previous chapter. This is per-haps easiest to see when there is a 'communication problem'.

Ben, for instance, was a 7 year old attending a school for young people with learning difficulties. He had no speech and was frequently aggressive towards people around him. The classroom assistant, Maureen, who worked with him for over a year found that his main channel of communication was smell. He greeted her every morning by smelling her clothes. Ben would never touch her, however, except in anger. In fact it seemed that being touched by others triggered his aggression. To establish a relationship with Ben, Maureen first of all used his main communication channel by always wearing the same strong perfume he seemed to like. She became increasingly sensitive to the signs that Ben was becoming anxious and was losing his temper and she was able to establish 'safe areas' with him away from the group, in particular on a red mat, where he knew he was safe and would become calm again. Over time Ben began to seek Maureen out each morning and greet her by smelling her clothing. Over time, too, she began to establish physical contact with Ben. She found that he would allow himself to be touched if he could control the touching by always having his hand over hers. It took six months before Maureen felt that they had a genuine relationship. Maureen was able slowly to become Ben's 'go-between' in increasingly making contact with others. He would allow himself to be touched through her. It was in this way that the physiotherapist was introduced to Ben and began forming a relationship with him.

Opening channels is first about relationships and secondly about listening in its broadest sense. It was through listening that Maureen was able to become sensitive to Ben's moods and feelings and was then able to use the safe areas to pre-empt his loss of temper. Listening is a major topic in its own right and is the focus of the next chapter.

In this section we shall be looking more specifically at opening up channels for people to express and explore their feelings, understandings and aspirations through reflecting on questions of the why, what and how of communication. In the answers to each there is an onus on the therapist to open possibilities of the reasons for, content of and ways of communicating.

Looking first towards reasons for communicating, the opening of channels is founded on openness about expectations. This requires therapists to be clear about their expectations of an open two-way flow of communication and mutuality in relationships, and conveying this to clients. Even when the therapist has such self-awareness, however, there can be barriers created by the expectations of the client. Dalton writes about the difficulties as a counsellor of people with communication problems:

> More difficult to approach . . . is the clients' conviction that what is wrong is physical and only physical. They see the practitioner as there to 'cure' the problem – to offer medicine, mechanical repair or exercises. Being asked about their feelings, about their views of themselves and their place in their worlds is experienced as an intrusion and this must be respected. (1994: 31)

She goes on to say:

> If the counsellor/therapist respects their wishes and works
> alongside them in their struggle for recovery, a degree of
> acceptance and understanding of their feelings that is at the
> heart of any counselling may be experienced. (1994: 32)

A similar statement could be made about the heart of the
human relations of helping in therapy. The opening up of
communication relies again, then, on the establishment of
the relationship. Why do people feel they can open up and
express their feelings, understandings and wishes? The answer
lies in a relationship of trust and mutual sensitivity – the type
of relationship described in the previous chapter.

Turning next to the question of what is communicated, there
can be barriers particularly to the expression of emotions.
Therapists work with people who are experiencing many different kinds of trauma in their lives: people who are experiencing physical illness and pain; people who are terminally ill;
people who have recently become disabled; people experiencing what Tschudin (1991) calls 'a moment of truth' in their
awareness of themselves and in their relationships with others;
and people experiencing radical changes in their style and
quality of life. These are contexts in which emotions can run
high: fear, anger and hostility, shock and guilt, grief and anxiety. How each individual acts and reacts depends on innumerable factors, including cultural differences and differences in
background and previous experiences. Two further general
points can be added to this picture. First, the therapist also
has emotional responses to therapeutic encounters, including
the general stresses and satisfactions of the job as well as
specific emotional responses towards the client and the client's experiences and feelings. Secondly, the communication
of emotions and interpersonal attitudes is generally fraught
with difficulties, including threats to self-esteem, misunder-
standings, denials and overreactions.

Opening up of what is communicated relies on the therapist
listening not only to what the client says but also to all those
non-verbal messages which have meaning in terms of the
client's feelings, understandings and wishes. This, in turn, is
grounded in the therapist's self-awareness of his feelings,

understandings and wishes. Returning to Maureen and, sub-sequently, the physiotherapist working with Ben, listening involved picking up signals – facial expressions, body pos-ture, noises – which indicated that Ben was about to become aggressive. It also involved learning, with Ben, what Maureen called 'his language of touch'. This was an idiosyncratic lan-guage with its own patterns and meanings. Maureen found, for instance, that Ben would use her hand to wipe off the touch, and possibly smell, of others.

Finally we turn to questions of how people communicate. Such questions are perhaps the most obvious in addressing the opening up of channels of communication: speech is only, for most people, the most obvious. Equally the most obvious barriers to communication are those which are seen as 'the client's communication problems'. There are many terms used to refer to and classify such problems, often beginning with the suffix 'dys', such as dysphasia, dyspraxia and dysarthria. Dysphasia is usually considered as having two forms: recep-tive, the impairment of comprehension of language, and expressive, the impairment of the expression of language. Dyspraxia and dysarthria refer to problems associated with the physical production of speech. This category of problems also includes any physical limitations to non-verbal commun-ication such as those effecting facial expressions, for instance in Parkinson's disease. At the most extreme, such barriers include a seeming total lack of communication, both verbal and non-verbal, as with some people in intensive care units.

Taking a broader perspective on communication, however, the difficulties of clients in expressing themselves is only part of the picture. It is important to reflect too on the channels through which therapists express their feelings, understand-ings and wishes. To take an obvious example, it can be useful for therapists to provide information in writing as well as verbal explanations. Secondly, the therapist may have 'communication problems', ranging from a lack of com-munication skills to one of the types of impairments men-tioned above. Thirdly, questions can be raised about the priority given to speech in communication. People can express themselves in many different ways which convey meaning as, or more, effectively than speech. This is true, of course, whether or not the client or the therapist has communication problems.

So what then are these other channels of communication which can be opened? The following list can only be indicative given that everything about us and everything we do carries the potential for communication.

1. The use of sign language is the clearest example of a communication mode or channel other than speech. Sign languages, as developed by deaf people, are actual languages with their own syntax as any other language. Clients may be either fluent in or use British Sign Language (or Makaton). The onus on therapists is the difficult task, if they are not fluent themselves, to learn what is essentially a foreign language, or at least use the services of a translator. It is important, too, not to make simplistic assumptions. There is a linguistic diversity among deaf people and there are also pros and cons to using translators. The book by Corker (1994) provides an excellent starting point for anyone seeking greater self-awareness and skills in this area.

2. Slightly less obvious, but no less important, is the use of translators generally. Though the therapist may have difficulties understanding the client, it is often the case that others, including other members of the client's family, other professionals or an advocate, are 'tuned in' to the client.

3. Writing is a mode of communication which is different from speech. Speech is of the moment, but writing can be more deliberate and intentional, and is more permanent, unless speech is recorded.

4. Dalton (1994: 28) suggests that other media of communication are essential when working with clients who have 'impaired communication': 'drawing and painting, materials which can be handled, and music and movement.' All of these can open communication whether or not the client would be said to have impaired communication. In particular, materials or toys of various kinds can be very useful when working with children using play. David, for instance, used play figures to talk over his anxieties

about returning to school after a lengthy illness. He used a set of plastic spiders which he had brought to a physiotherapy session to set up a pretend school which he then attacked with some larger play figures. This play scene which was initiated and controlled by David provided a context in which he could disclose his concerns. Joining children in their play is an effective way of opening channels of communication.

5. Photographs can also be a useful key to opening two-way communication. For instance, I interviewed a woman with learning difficulties in her home with the aim of recording her story of how she came to leave an institution where she had spent many years, get married and live, with some support, in a flat of her own. She told me her story in fits and starts until she got out her photograph album. At this point she became motivated and articulate in her explanations of the people, events and circumstances in each picture.

6. A 'language of touch' was referred to above in relation to Ben. Touch can convey messages, sometimes subtle and sometimes obvious, which go beyond words.

7. Finally in this short list, we must include facial expressions and gesture. At their simplest such signals suggest negative or positive feelings towards people, events or experiences. With clients who have profound impairments, expressions of discrimination and preferences can be the basic level of communication with which the therapist needs to be receptive.

This chapter closes with a quote from Dalton (1994: 30) which she applies to counsellors, but which can be applied to all therapists: 'The counsellor needs to be inventive and to encourage experimentation in clients, who may find they have resources within themselves that have never before been tapped.'

Personal reflections 6.1

In previous chapters, suggestions for 'Personal Reflections' have attempted to convey the challenges that human relations of helping can pose for the therapist. Reflecting on communication exerts similar challenges in the questioning of beliefs, feelings, thinking and actions, but also extra challenges in that acts of communication are transitory and happen between people. A major part of this is the challenge of noticing what goes unnoticed. How might you, then reflect on communication?

1. The easiest approach is to attempt to observe and record communication either during or immediately after an interaction. There are a number of different ways to do this which vary from the least to the most systematic.

    (a) The least systematic involves making notes about anything you see as significant in the client's expression of his thinking or feeling. Making notes during an interaction or 'session' can be more immediate and less distorted by memory, but can also interfere with the interaction itself. It is difficult to listen and make notes at the same time.

    (b) Being more systematic involves preparing yourself with lists of the sorts of things you could watch for. This could include lists of behaviours which are either general, such as facial expressions, or more specific, such as smiling, and also lists of emotions and thoughts that might be expressed.

    (c) The most systematic approaches involve checklists, which can be useful, for instance, when working with people who are profoundly and multiply impaired. A good example is the Affective Communication Assessment (Coupe et al., 1988) which has a highly detailed list of possible movements of the client together with spaces for interpreting the meaning of the movements.

2. Make a video of yourself working with a client. Videos have the advantage of being a permanent record which can be replayed repeatedly. They, of course, raise practical and ethical problems, ranging from the simple access to a camera to the 'informed consent' of the client. Furthermore, there are difficulties in that the presence of a video camera changes the situation. You

and the client may feel self-conscious and actually behave differently because you are being filmed. Nevertheless, because of the transitory nature of communication, video recording can be an extremely valuable technique of observation which can provide the therapist with insights into many of the messages he is not aware of during interactions. Approaches to analysing videos can again vary in terms of how systematic you are, as above.

3. A third possible approach to observing communication is to invite a third person to be present as an observer. The difficulties are the same as those involved in video recording. The advantages are those of working with a partner: the insights offered by a critical friend.

7

Listening

Are you sitting comfortably?

'Are you sitting comfortably?' seems an apt phrase to introduce a chapter on listening. It was used to introduce the 'Listen With Mother' radio programme of story-time for young children. It reminds us, first, that listening is more than hearing. To listen we have to attend and, hence, the question of being comfortable.

Yet listening is more than this. In a broader sense it is more than attending to the spoken word. Deaf people listen. As we saw in Chapter 6, messages about how the other person is feeling are often conveyed non-verbally. Yet it is more than this too. Listening includes listening to ourselves, our own understanding of and feelings about the messages the other person is sending. Furthermore, listening is part of interaction and a two-way flow of communication. Part of listening is the messages sent by the listener to indicate that she is attending, or not, and understanding, or not, the messages being sent.

However, it is even more than this. There is a quality to the whole listening process which takes it beyond being a set of skills or processes in communication. This was reflected in an early study by Mayo (1933) whose work suggested that when we are listened to by someone who is truly understanding, who takes the trouble to listen to us as we consider our problem and who acts on what we say, that experience can change our whole outlook on the world. There is little wonder, then, that people have found the actual word 'listening'

inadequate, as it sounds so mundane and such an easy process that we do not really have to think about it. The term
'active listening' is often used in an attempt to capture the full
complexities and indicate that it is not a passive process. The
Chinese listening symbol (Figure 7.1) gives a far fuller picture. It is much more challenging and gives a better notion of
the processes we shall be exploring in this chapter. Using
this Chinese character as a basis for definition, listening is: a
process in which *I* give my *ears, eyes* and *heart* in *undivided
attention* to *you*. When it is thought of like this, listening is
not just hearing, it is an intense personal involvement with
another person. It is something we learn, rather than something we either can or cannot do, and learning requires
self-reflection.

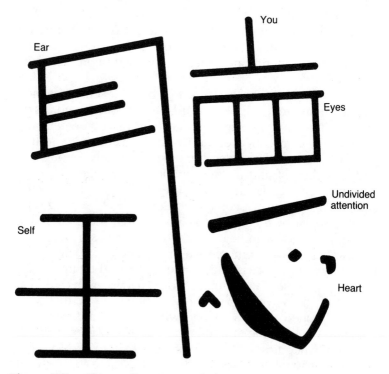

Figure 7.1   *Chinese listening symbol*

Personal reflections 7.1

The purpose of this exercise is to help you look at your skills in actively listening to others. One good way to do this is to make an audio recording of yourself talking with another person. If possible work again with your partner. Make a recording of the person talking about herself. The following are some guidelines:

1. You will of course need the permission of the person with whom you choose to talk. You may also need to consult others if, for instance, you are going to talk to a young person. If you are working with your partner, you will already have gone through these preliminary discussions.
2. There are some technical questions you will need to consider. Try out your tape-recorder first! You will also need to consider the location of your recording: will there be interruptions? One person doing this exercise left the tape-recorder too near a noisy radiator.

Listen carefully to the tape: listen to yourself rather than your partner. Listen with your partner and ask her opinion. Make a few notes on the following:

1. How do you use questions? The most common mistake in this type of exercise is to use far too many questions and to ask closed questions which can be answered in a word or two.
2. Do you leave silences? Another common mistake is to jump in as soon as the other person hesitates.
3. Do you ever reflect back to the person the ideas or feelings being communicated to you?
4. Overall, do you think you are helping the person talk about what she wants to talk about . . . or what you want to hear about? Did your partner feel she could talk freely and openly with you and that you helped her say what she wanted to say?

Listening is not as easy as many of us would like to think. You might find it useful to make a second tape along the same lines as the first one, when you have read about all the listening skills we examine in this chapter.

Like talking to a brick wall

An exercise commonly used to start people thinking about listening involves working in pairs. During the first part of the activity one person talks about a topic she has chosen while the other does all she can to show that she is focusing herself completely on what the speaker is saying, doing and meaning by her words and behaviour. The listener then summarizes in her own words to the other person what has been said, and finally the speaker reports back from her side about how well she feels she has been listened to. This is repeated by the pair exchanging roles, so that the person who has been listening now becomes the speaker. However, the other person this time has to do all she can to show that she is not listening. This causes much laughter over the frustrations of the speakers and the antics of the non-listeners, such as fidgeting and pretending to look out of the window. One person even removed her shoe and started banging it on the table, as if to remove a stone. In the discussions afterwards, people have talked about feelings such as resentment, anger, inadequacy and diminished self-esteem, but they also agree that 'talking to a brick wall' is a frequent occurrence in their daily lives. They easily recognize situations they have experienced in which there was little two-way communication.

Two conclusions are drawn in these discussions. The first is that effective communication is both rare and difficult. Much so-called 'communication' involves each person airing her views: while the other person talks, the 'listener' is busy formulating her next contribution to the conversation. The second conclusion is that not listening is an aggressive or manipulative act and not being listened to can be an emotionally debilitating experience in which the self is demeaned and denied.

A starting point for reflection on ourselves as listeners, then, is all those barriers which build brick walls between people and pre-empt any two-way flow of communication. There are many such bricks. Figure 7.2 is drawn largely from discussions with students (see also Bolton, 1979), to show the potential bricks in the wall. From the outset it is essential to remember

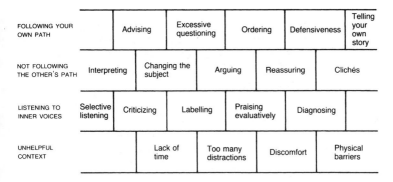

FOLLOWING YOUR OWN PATH		Advising	Excessive questioning		Ordering	Defensiveness	Telling your own story
NOT FOLLOWING THE OTHER'S PATH	Interpreting		Changing the subject	Arguing		Reassuring	Clichés
LISTENING TO INNER VOICES	Selective listening	Criticizing		Labelling	Praising evaluatively	Diagnosing	
UNHELPFUL CONTEXT			Lack of time	Too many distractions		Discomfort	Physical barriers

Figure 7.2 *Like talking to a brick wall*

that the biggest brick in the wall is the belief that it is other people who build walls and not ourselves. As listening is achieved by people together, so is the building of walls.

Unhelpful context

The first layer of bricks in the wall is an unhelpful context. Active listening requires a space to give undivided attention: a space of time, place and mind which is free, or relatively so, from all those distractions from within as well as from without. There is no attention to give if it is invested elsewhere. Lack of time is the most often quoted barrier, by professionals at least. The listener's attention is focused on another pressing appointment and her own need to limit the encounter: the 'such-a-busy-man' syndrome as I have heard it called.

Other bricks in the wall of bad listening are often built on lack of time, such as selective listening, reassuring and advising. When time is felt to be pressing, for instance, it is quicker to offer a word or two of reassurance than to allow the other person to talk through her difficulties. As usual it is more easily recognized from the receiving end, from experiences for instance of trying to talk to someone who is continually looking at her watch. One student wrote in her journal about her appointments with her line manager who sat behind his desk and continued to work on other things throughout. He would be looking through his papers and even writing while she tried to talk about pressing concerns. In her journal she wrote of frustration, anger and, above all, 'feeling small'. She did find a strategy for coping with this: she simply stopped talking whenever his attention was diverted and, in this case, it worked.

From the side of the would-be listener, lack of time is often too easily rationalized. In a busy day, giving more time to one person can mean less time with another. It is impossible to have rules which will cover every situation, but there are some principles which can be useful.

1. Be sure that however short the length of time, it is given in undivided attention, as in the Chinese character, to the other person. Whenever possible this requires 'a deep breath', both literally and in the mind, to put into abeyance physical and mental stress of time pressures (see below).
2. If insufficient time is available tell the other person how long you have got, or find out how long they have got, and agree at the outset on what will be covered in that time.
3. When necessary, agree that there is insufficient time and arrange another meeting.

There are other important bricks in this foundation layer of the wall: too many distractions, discomfort and physical barriers. Sometimes solutions can be quick and easy, such as a rearrangement of the seating, so that you are not separated by a desk, or by retiring to a quieter room. Some solutions are more long term, such as redecorating or refurbishing a room. It is important to remember, though, the inner as well as the outer, physical environment. Some people, for instance, are more comfortable talking in a busy working environment than a quiet side room. What is a 'helpful context' depends on the whole situation of who is involved, what is being talked about and why.

Listening to inner voices

This may seem a strange layer of bricks: good listening involves listening to the inner voice. The inner voice builds the wall when it is so loud it distorts, devalues and drowns the voice of the other person. It is a natural tendency to make judgements about other people and the messages they are sending. It is a natural tendency, too, to put your own point of view forward: 'to put in your own two-pennorth'. You may have overheard, or indeed remember being part of, conversations in which each person is doing no more than speaking to her own concerns and interests. These bricks have been labelled: selective listening, criticizing, labelling, praising evaluatively and diagnosing. Each is a violation on the voice of the other person which can channel the flow of conversation towards the judgements of the listener.

Criticizing is the inner judgemental voice of approval or disapproval. It can begin before a word is spoken. Judgements can begin from the way a person is dressed, make-up, hairstyle, gait, jewellery and so on. Deep-seated values, beliefs and prejudices can be a screen to listening to the individual. This is perhaps easiest to see in areas which can arouse high passions, such as physical violence, child abuse and drug-taking. In some situations it is possible for the listener to put her judgements in abeyance and in some situations, too, they can be reflected on and challenged by listening to the other person. Nevertheless, preconceptions and feelings can be so strong that criticism is an impenetrable barrier to listening.

Labelling and diagnosing are ways of categorizing people which can devalue them and what they are saying. Labelling can be seen as a form of criticism, a set of presumptions, prejudgements and prejudices about a supposed type or stereotype of person. The other person is not an individual in her own right, but a type of person. There are, of course, many such labels: aggressive, chauvinist, disabled, deaf, and so on, including derogatory, name-calling labels. It is not that labels are wrong in themselves. Indeed, they can be used to affirm positive identity ('Black is beautiful') and bring people together to challenge the discrimination and abuse they experience. In the context of these discussion, however, labelling can be a barrier to listening to another person as a unique individual.

Diagnosis does involve listening, but a form of technical listening to pick up clues about conclusions being drawn (see 'Assessment' in Chapter 4). It might be conclusions, for instance, that the other person is under stress or deceiving herself. Everything the other person says and does is sifted for signs to confirm the diagnosis. As you may have noted, labelling and diagnosing are part of the processes of therapy. The dilemma for therapists is that the techniques involved can thwart listening, as conveyed in the Chinese listening symbol.

Listening is not just internal to the listener – it is built into the whole two-way flow of communication. The inner voice can direct and subvert this flow. In selective listening, only part of what the other person says and does is being responded to. One version of this is evaluative praise. This can be seen as a subtle manipulation of communication. To be positive towards the other person can encourage her and help her have confidence in herself and what she is saying. When such praise is dictated by the inner voice, however, it is selective and given in accordance to the listener's judgements of what is important, right and required. It then becomes a dam in the flow of communication.

Not following the other's path

The brick wall builds layer by layer. The foundations for not following the other's path have been laid in the previous layers of bricks. In general, these are ways of responding which block, divert, distort and rechannel the track the other person is on. Interpreting builds directly on listening to inner voices. It is directing the flow of conversation in accordance with the listener's judgements and diagnosis about the other person and what she is saying. To tell the other person that she is being defensive, for instance, may actually make the other person become defensive, or change the subject to talking about the other person's supposed defensiveness.

Changing the subject is simply switching the conversation from the other person's to your own concerns. In discussing this in a seminar, one student spoke vehemently and passionately about her husband, who it seemed to her was constantly changing the subject. She felt he dominated conversations and denied her concerns. This can arise in many ways, again the earlier layers providing the foundations. One source is avoidance, as seemingly with the student's husband, of emotionally difficult concerns, such as death, sickness and personal conflicts.

Argument is a fairly obvious brick. You may, for instance, be able to think of conversations in which one person blamed the other person and took up a position or argued just for the sake of it, without real beliefs or feelings. More subtly, as with changing the subject, rational argument can deny or distract from strong feelings and emotions of the other person by getting away from personal issues.

Reassurance can also be a denial of strengths of feelings. The rushed few words of support may be an attempt to show caring, but can be a means of closing down communication. Clichés are a form of reassurance: 'Time's a great healer', 'You've got to take the rough with the smooth', or 'Let bygones be bygones'. Such stock platitudes avoid rather than reflect the particular concerns of the other person.

Following your own path

In general terms, this layer of the brick wall involves the 'listener' taking over and dominating the flow of conversation. Instead of helping the other person explore her concerns and decide on her own directions, her needs and solutions are decided for her. These bricks have been labelled: advising, excessive questioning, ordering, defensiveness and telling your own story.

So why is advising a brick in this wall blocking communication? It can be seen as a way of helping rather than a barrier to communication. In providing help, therapists are looked towards for advice. It becomes a barrier when stock advice pre-empts listening. It is easy to provide solutions without really knowing the problem. There are two dangers. First, the advice may be rejected because it does not fit the person's particular problem and it is not *her* solution. Equally dangerous, is the possibility that the advice may be followed religiously, as it is seen as coming from the expert, and whether the solution works or not she may be quickly back for another 'shot of advice' which she can come to rely on to provide solutions.

Ordering is a form of advising backed with authority: 'You'll have to live with the consequences if you don't comply.' Such threats do not have to be explicit, but can be inherent in people's perceptions of therapy. The dangers are those of advising generally, but 'writ large'.

In the 'Personal reflections 7.1' it was suggested that you record yourself in an encounter with another person. This exercise has been used with teachers, asking them to help pupils talk about themselves and their experiences in schools. In many cases, two things emerge when the contributions of the teachers are listened to: there are no silences; and each teacher asks a string of closed-ended questions. At the worst extreme, it is an interrogation and the young person slowly stumbles to a halt, increasingly responding only to the questions and increasingly answering with single words or short phrases. The conversation, if it can be called such, ends when the teacher runs out of questions.

Telling your own story, which is a form of self-disclosure, is a brick which is often named by people when talking about the wall, seemingly from heartfelt experiences. It is responses which say 'done that, been there' and the 'listener' launches into her own narrative. The positive messages are obvious. It can be a way of saying: 'I'm with you. I understand.' It can help the other person talk by recognizing her concerns as being legitimate. Telling your own story can be a brick in the wall, however, in two ways. First, it can deny the individuality of experiences. For instance, the listener's experiences and feelings of grief following a death in the family will be quite different from those of the other person. Grief is an individual experience. Telling your own story can devalue the experiences and feelings of the other person as being common. At an extreme, the listener does not have to listen because she supposedly knows what the other person has been through. Secondly, perhaps more obviously, it is the 'listener' who is dominating and being listened to. Telling your own story simply denies the other person space to tell hers.

Defensiveness has been named as a separate brick, though it can underlie this whole layer of the wall. Excessive questioning, advising, ordering and telling your own story can all be expressions of the listener's defensiveness. They can be ways of putting up a professional, expert or knowledgeable screen which promotes and establishes the credentials of the listener. All the baggage of training, accountability, appraisal and professional responsibility can help cement the wall with defensiveness.

Personal reflections 7.2

Concentrate, in your journal, writing on yourself as a listener. Look at any event or interaction you have recorded in terms of 'talking to a brick wall'. Can you find examples of bricks you built in the other person's path?

Dismantling the wall

This idea of talking to a brick wall has been built layer by layer because it is all too easy to get a simplistic picture of being a good listener. Listening is a challenging and soul-searching process in which the listener not only meets the other person but also meets herself. There is no simple set of rules by which you can become a more effective listener. Listening is constructed in each encounter between people. The good listener not only shares the experiences and feelings of the other person, she confronts her own beliefs and emotions, reflects her understanding back to the other person, and the other person experiences 'good listening' and reflects this back to the listener. This is a meeting of hearts and minds, not in agreement, but in sharing through a two-way flow of communication. We are moving on to look at ways or possibilities of 'dismantling the wall', but such possibilities are meaningless unless they are drawn through your 'Personal reflections' into your work as a therapist with other people (Table 7.1).

Table 7.1 *Dismantling the wall*

Being with the other person	Following the other person's concerns	Reflecting the other person's concerns
Square	Openers	Paraphrasing
Open	Encouragers	Reflecting feeling
Lean	Questions	Reflecting listener's feelings
Eye contact	Silence	Reflecting meaning
Relax		Summarizing
	Context	
	Awareness	
	Presence	

Being with the other person

Listening, when there is face-to-face contact, is founded on being with the other person both physically and mentally. This is often called 'attending', though as usual the word seems inadequate for conveying the intensity of involvement which is better conveyed by the Chinese symbol. Directing your self, ears, eyes and heart in undivided attention to the other person begins even before the actual encounter. As mentioned above, it starts by clearing the mind of distractions and worries and a putting of judgements into abeyance. This has been called by Kottler and Kottler (1993: 39) a 'cleansing breath': 'A deep breath helps clear yourself of muddled and distracting thoughts and helps "centre" yourself on the interaction that is about to begin.'

In exercises in which students identify and discuss what a good listener does, five behaviours are named which coincide with Egan's (1990) idea of SOLER. This is a mnemonic to help people remember five features of a posture of involvement. We show we are listening just as much by what we do as what we say. It is easy to see this by thinking of people who do not listen to you. You 'know' they are not listening to you.

1. A good listener tends to face the other person. She faces the other person Squarely. A person who is not listening is sometimes said to 'give the cold shoulder'.

2. Maintaining an Open position with no barriers of desk, crossed arms, etc., is an important part of involvement.
3. We also can think the other person is listening more closely to us when they Lean towards us.
4. Eye contact can, of course, be highly important. At its simplest this can involve being at the same eye level so that the listener is not looking down on the speaker, but communication through eye contact is never simple. The eyes can be a 'window on the soul' to get inside the other person's skin and understand her experiences from her perspective. Eye contact is one the most intimate ways of relating with others. However, as with each of these postures of involvement, the meaning of eye contact is in the eye of the beholder. Eye contact can be interpreted in many ways, depending on context. It can convey attentiveness and interest in the other person, but eye contact can also be intrusive, embarrassing and even threatening.

   This can also be problematic if the client or therapist has a visual impairment. Sally French, who is herself a physiotherapist and is visually impaired, says: 'I know eye-contact is very important but this is something which is often used as a way of excluding visually impaired people from work involving counselling and communication which I don't think is justified. . . . I know from experience that it *is* a problem but I don't think it is unsurmountable especially if one is open and honest about it and then the other person understands and adjusts to it' (1994: personal communication).
5. A good listener tends to be Relaxed. We have all been through the frustrating experience of trying to talk to someone who seems to have no time and thinks she should be somewhere else.

Though the SOLER formula is useful, it is insufficient on its own. It is possible to do all of these without really listening and without the other person feeling that she is being listened to. SOLER can be only a posture of involvement without a psychological involvement. A second set of factors in being with another person can be added to the SOLER formula. They can be given the appropriate mnemonic CAP.

The first factor is Context. At the most straightforward level this refers to a non-distracting environment: non-distracting in that the physical, social and psychological bricks in the wall have been removed. At another level, Context is what gives the SOLER behaviours meaning, that is, the context of the two-way flow of communication. As pointed out earlier, eye contact can send messages which are quite contrary to those of attending to and being with the other person: eye contact can express threat and intrusion. To give another example, being relaxed can send messages of lack of concern or disinterest, or in other words being too 'laid back'. To put it succinctly, SOLER behaviours only promote being with the other person if the other person actually feels that she has the listener's undivided attention.

Which takes us to our second factor: Awareness. This is a self-awareness by the listener of her own body and behaviour as a source of communication. Such awareness comes from two directions: from within in the continuous monitoring by the listener of her own feelings and responses towards the other person, such as feelings of anxiety or lack of acceptance; and from without in the continuous monitoring of the other person's response to the listener. As Nelson-Jones (1982: 334) says: 'The basis for listening to others is to be able to listen accurately to oneself.'

The third feature is probably the most important yet the most difficult to define: Presence. As usual, it is the lack of presence which is easier to recognize, as signified by 'a glossing over of the eyes.' The listener may use all the SOLER behaviours but still not be with the other person. They are psychologically removed and might even be jerked back by the question, 'Are you listening to me?' The following set of questions (adapted from Egan, 1990: 111) are useful for listeners to ask of themselves in monitoring the quality of their presence with the other person:

- What values are operative in this interaction?
- What are my attitudes towards this particular person?
- Am I experiencing some kind of conflict in terms of my values or attitudes right now? Am I indifferent to the other person and what she is saying?

- How would I rate the quality of my presence to the other person right now?
- How are my values and attitudes being expressed in what I am saying to the other person?
- How are my values and attitudes being expressed in my non-verbal behaviour, including eye contact, tone of voice, movements and so on?
- How might I be more effectively present to this person?

Following the other person's concerns

The goal of listening is not just being with the other person, though this is the essential foundation, but also to journey with the other person through her experiences and feelings. Following the other person's concerns involves helping her talk about whatever she wants to talk about, rather than what you want to talk about or hear. This includes: staying out of the other person's way as she discovers and explores her own views, feelings and needs, by not proffering advice, being judgemental or, in other words, building the wall; picking up meaning and understanding of the other person's world and experiences from her viewpoint, so you can discover how she views the situation in her terms rather than yours; encouraging and facilitating the other person in her exploration.

We shall look at four ways of following the other person's concerns: openers, encouragers, questions and silence.

Openers

Bolton (1979) calls these 'door openers' and they are unforceful, open invitations to talk. Basically you are saying: 'I'm interested in hearing about it.' What to say specifically depends on the context. It can involve:

- a description of the other person's body language, e.g. 'You're looking a bit down'
- an invitation to talk, e.g. 'How have things gone for you today?'

- silence, waiting for the other person to speak
- eye contact.

There are of course problems: if only it was so easy to open doors of communication! Such openers may be useless with young children, people who have blocked off from talking about their concerns, and indeed in any situation in which communication is difficult, whether the difficulty comes from the listener, the other person, or both. There can, however, be other ways of opening the door. For instance, with young children it is important to enter the child's world by joining her play.

Another frequently mentioned problem is that the other person seems to 'beat around the bush': talking about anything and everything other than what seems central to her immediate concerns. This can be defensiveness and also a testing out of the relationship: is the listener open and trustworthy? In some situations it can be necessary to go on to challenge the other person, for instance by reflecting that you feel there is something bothering her, but she seems to have problems opening up about it. Challenging in this way can be problematic and may suppress the other person even further. It is usually better not to pressurize the other person, certainly until a good relationship has been established.

The most frequently mentioned problem in discussions with students was put succinctly by one person: 'You can open up a can of worms.' There are two dimensions to this. Some problems are so emotionally charged and value-ridden that the listener finds it extremely difficult or impossible to be open. The second related dimension is the listener's feelings of being powerless to help. There are questions here for therapists as to where their sphere of responsibility ends. It is essential to remember that there are other possible sources of help and, in particular, that the therapist is *not* a counsellor. There are situations in which the other person has to be referred elsewhere for help. This is not to suggest that referral is always a straightforward solution or an easy option. It can be a real dilemma for therapists, and any professionals, who take a client-centred approach and believe that they are concerned with the 'person-as-a-whole'.

Encouragers

These are the head-nods, 'Mm-hm's, 'Oh?'s, 'And?'s, etc., which encourage the speaker to keep telling you her story in her own way. Such little encouragers say: 'Keep talking. I'm with you.' As Munro *et al.* (1983) point out, minimal encouragers are effective in keeping the client talking, whereas too much talking by the therapist leaves no space. There are dangers even in such a seemingly simple technique. They can be used by the listener, often unconsciously, to direct the conversation towards her own agenda. This happens through a selective use of encouragers, that is, the listener is being more encouraging when the other person is talking about what the listener wants to hear about.

Infrequent questions

When students have made audio tapes of themselves talking with clients, the most common mistake is to ask too many questions. The conversation becomes more like an interview or even an interrogation. Good listeners tend to ask fewer questions; the questions follow the concerns of the other person; and the questions are open, i.e. not just looking for one word answers. (We shall be looking at questioning in some detail in the next chapter.)

Silence

Finally, people can be helped to talk by the listener simply waiting for them to say something. Silence is crucial to following the other person's concerns: as the old saying goes, 'The beginning of wisdom is silence'. It provides space for the other person, and the listener, to think and reflect. Silence is a way of keeping out of the other person's way.

Many people, however, do not like silences. They tend to feel uncomfortable and jump in and say something themselves rather than waiting for other people to speak. Silence can be embarrassing for the listener and threatening for the other person. Indeed a distinction can be made between 'embarrassed silence' and 'attentive silence'.

Openers, encouragers, questions and silence only have meaning in context. They can only be part of following the other person's concerns if the other person feels the listener is providing space, understanding her viewpoint and encouraging her to explore. Awareness continues to be crucial as the listener reflects on what the other person means and on her own emotions and feelings being raised. The quality of presence is also essential in following the other person's concerns, otherwise listening will be, at best, superficial. Following the path of the other person is not a passive act of 'being led', but requires the listener to be an active co-traveller on the journey.

Reflecting the other person's concerns

As emphasized earlier, listening must be considered as part of the two-way flow of communication. Good listening involves not only understanding the other person's experiences and feelings, but also demonstrating to the other person that she is being understood and accepted. Reflecting can communicate understanding to the other person and, from the listener's side, checks understanding. Understanding can be seen as a guessing process.

Language is imprecise and non-verbal communication is even more ephemeral. Furthermore, as mentioned above, people often talk about safe topics, such as the weather, rather than broaching real concerns. Indeed, we sometimes do not know what we think or feel until we have talked it over with someone who is really listening. The mirror that a good listener provides aids self-awareness and self-understanding. Reflection also helps the listener concentrate on what is actually being expressed: not what she is expecting, would like to hear, or the noise in her own thoughts and feelings. It is, then, a major part of building listening and dismantling the wall. We shall be looking at five ways of reflecting: paraphrasing, summative reflections, reflecting feelings, reflecting the listener's feelings and reflecting meaning.

Paraphrasing

This is simply the skill of telling the person what she has just said in your own words. The listener repeats the essence of what the other person has said. This is not a repeating back of the speaker's words, parrot fashion. The listener reflects back what the speaker has said using the listener's own words, but without distorting what has been expressed. This can sound a stilted and artificial thing to do, and can feel as such when you are first trying to do this. However, when it is done well it is simply a natural part of the flow of conversation and can be extremely useful in showing the person that you are listening carefully and help you check that you have understood what has been said. Paraphrasing can also be like breathing spaces in which the other person can think through what she will say next.

Summative reflections

This is a brief restatement of ideas and feelings that the speaker has expressed over a longer period of conversation. It helps the speaker see what you have understood from what has been said. Again it is essential that this is done without distortion. When it is selective it can help focus the person on the main concerns and can give a sense of movement in the conversation. It can help in the movement from one stage to another in the use of counselling skills in therapy, for instance when moving towards specifying clear goals. As with other kinds of reflection, this can become a process of challenging when it is demanding on the other person, for instance in clarifying the focus of the person's main concerns.

Reflecting feelings

Feelings are not always expressed in words. They are more often conveyed by what the person does, facial expression, posture, eyes etc. In fact, we tend to believe these signals more than we believe what people say. For example, if some-one tells you she is 'feeling all right' and at the same time she is frowning, wringing her hands and looking down, you will tend to think that she is really not 'feeling all right'. The reverse is true, too, of course. The therapist will tend to be distrusting of a client who says she is in constant pain but whose general posture and mobility suggest otherwise. It is not easy, however, accurately to reflect back feelings of which perhaps even the other person is only half aware. It needs the sort of listening shown in the Chinese symbol in Figure 7.1.

Reflecting the listener's feelings

This form of reflection is somewhat anomalous to the mirror of physical movement that there can be between speaker and listener. It requires 'being in tune' with each other so that the feelings that the listener is picking up inside herself will actually aid the other person towards self-understanding. The listener is reflecting back by sharing her own feelings from what has been expressed: 'It really makes me feel sad when you say that . . . ' or 'I feel confused by what you are saying . . .'. This helps towards a two-way flow. Both can feel that they are truly sharing feelings. This is a difficult thing to do and requires a high level of genuineness and empathy if the listener's rather than the speaker's feelings are not to dominate the conversation.

Reflecting meaning

This is perhaps the most difficult of all the different processes of reflection to do accurately. It is not only a reflection of the feelings being expressed, but links these to the speaker's experiences, action or understanding. Thus, such reflections often take the form of, 'You feel . . . because . . .' statements. For instance, 'You feel guilty because you've had so much time off work and you feel you're letting others down.' If there is not an open two-way flow of communication and empathy has not been established, there are obvious dangers. It may be that the listener's reflections put ideas into the other person's head which direct and manipulate the speaker into the listener's presumptions, expectations, concerns and interests. Or it may be that the other person thinks the listener has totally misunderstood, but for one reason or another does not correct the listener. Accurate reflection of meaning, however, can be a real help to the other person in exploring, becoming aware of and understanding her experiences, feelings, concerns and, indeed, herself.

If anything, Context, Awareness and Presence become even more important in accurate reflection. This is because of the dangers of distortion, misdirection and manipulation in the communication process. Reflection of meaning is sometimes referred to as advanced empathy. Reflection becomes advanced empathy when it accurately goes beyond what is directly expressed to what is implied: 'reading between the lines'. Context is crucial in that there is a subtle and complex interplay of reflections on reflections and feedback on feedback. The accuracy of reflections can only be judged in the context of the continuing two-way flow of communication. At its simplest this can be a direct positive ('Yes you're right, that's why I feel like that') or negative statement, but more usually it is implicit in the move towards self-exploration and self-understanding. The importance of awareness is also evident. The accuracy of reflections depends not only on the listener's awareness of the other person's feelings but also of her own feelings. This is crucial to the two-way flow of communication and the establishment of genuineness and empathy. Finally, accurate reflection would simply be impossible without presence on the part of the listener. If presence in following the other's path means being an active co-traveller, in reflecting it is accurately comparing maps on the journey through the other person's concerns.

Personal reflections 7.3

1. As in 'Personal reflections 7.2' concentrate in your journal writing on yourself as a listener. This time look at events or interactions in terms of 'dismantling the brick wall'. Can you pick out points at which you used any of the skills in Table 7.1?
2. Another way of learning the skills of listening is to practise them in safe and secure circumstances, preferably with partners who will work with you through the exercises. If possible work with your partner, but it would be

useful to have a third person present who could act as an observer.

(a) This activity is designed to make you more aware of what you do when listening. As the listener you should try to pay attention to the speaker. Encourage the speaker to keep talking and make it clear that you are listening, *without using words.* The speaker should talk for three minutes on one of the following topics:

- the best thing that happened to me last week
- the things I like or dislike about my job
- my favourite hobby.

(b) The listener should reflect back to the speaker everything she has 'heard', including the responses to non-verbal as well as verbal messages.

(c) The speaker should reflect back to the listener what the experience of being listened to was like. The sort of questions that can be covered are:

- was the speaker able to share experiences, feelings and understandings?
- how well did the listener attend?
- what were the listener's thoughts, feelings and sensations throughout?
- at what points was the listener genuine, at what points did she show warmth or empathy?
- this particular exercise concentrates on the non-verbal messages of the listener – what difference did this make to the experiences of the speaker and listener?

3. This second activity for practising listening skills essentially repeats an exercise in Chapter 4. This time, however, you are asked to concentrate on the listening skills being employed. The speaker should think of an unresolved problem in her life. The listener should apply the stages of a counselling process to work with the other person through:

(a) defining the problem
(b) re-evaluating the problem
(c) her aims and goals in solving the problem

(d) an assessment of the relevant opportunities and personal resources

(e) an action plan of what she proposes to do

(f) how she intends to evaluate the results of her efforts.

The helper should use all the skills of active listening in:

(a) attending

(b) following

(c) reflecting

the thoughts and feelings of the other person.

The helper and speaker, and observer if possible, should then go through the steps (b) and (c) of activity 2 above.

Chapter

8

Challenging

What is 'challenging'?

The term 'challenging' is used here to mean a process of demanding or helping others make demands of themselves. As Egan states:

> Put most simply, challenging is an invitation to examine internal or external behaviour that seems to be self-defeating, harmful to others, or both and to change the behaviour if it is found to be so. (1990: 184)

Such self-defeating behaviours can take many forms, including reactions of helplessness to perceived failure: such as blaming stable qualities of the self, such as a supposed lack of ability, rather than temporary factors that can be overcome, such as lack of motivation. Attempting to help someone see that he could be successful if he tried harder or simply tried again is a common form of challenging which you may recognize from your own experiences, particularly if you are a parent.

Challenging, then, facilitates changes in thinking, feeling or action. It is a process of re-evaluation and reorientation and can involve anything from taking new information into account to changing whole life-views. Clients undertaking therapy are often in a transition phase of their life. They are experiencing changes of many kinds, sometimes quite traumatic upheavals in their whole quality and style of life. But challenging can and should be thought of as a two-way process. It is part of reflective practice:

> To create change, then, we must examine our own behaviours carefully, bring unexamined assumptions to awareness and consciously self-monitor both our behaviour and our assumptions. (Osterman and Kottkamp, 1993: 20)

In general terms, challenging can be seen as an extension of reflection. To separate 'listening' from 'challenging' is solely a matter of convenience. They are both part of furthering human relations in helping, and the principles discussed in Chapter 4 apply equally to both. Thus we already have a basis for thinking about the concept of challenging which can be summarized as follows.

- challenging is part of the whole process of building and maintaining self-awareness, effective relationships and two-way communication
- challenging builds on listening: attending, following and reflecting
- challenging is guided by the principles which apply to all human relations in helping
- as a part of reflection, challenging demands a re-examination of thinking, feeling and behaviour and those demands are self-generated in dialogue with others
- challenging which is not an integral part of the human relations of helping can be the cornerstone of a wall between the therapist and the client.

One way of looking at the skills or strategies which can be employed in challenging is in relation to their main focus. A starting point for thinking about challenging is in terms of the demands being made for re-evaluating thinking, feeling and action. Five focal points can be identified (Table 8.1):

1. *Information* – the focus here is the 'facts' or 'concepts' which underpin a person's understanding of a situation.
2. *Client's concerns* – the focus here is the actual process of focusing at any stage of therapy, including on problems and solutions.

Table 8.1   *Challenging*

Focus for challenging/demands	*Strategies for helping*
Information	Begin with what is already known
	Present the information
	Check the result
	Ensure retention
Client's concerns	Summative reflections
	Concreteness
Relationships and communication	Immediacy
Client's self-awareness	Reflecting feelings
	Advanced empathy
	Confrontation
Therapist's self awareness	Self-disclosure/sharing
	<u>C</u>ontext
	<u>A</u>wareness
	<u>P</u>resence

3. *Relationships and communication* – the focus here is the human relations of helping, particularly the relationship and communication between the client and the therapist.
4. *Client's self-awareness* – the focus here is the client's understandings, experiences and feelings.
5. *Therapist's self-awareness* – the focus here is the therapist's understandings, experiences and feelings.

Information

Perhaps the most common way of challenging for therapists is providing a client with new information. Davis (1993) suggests a list of stages in providing information which seems to comply with the approach to challenging we are taking here. There are four stages.

1. Begin with what he already knows

Information has meaning in terms of the person's existing understanding. It is all too easy to provide information which is incomprehensible, irrelevant, useless and even inaccessible. In a way this is a 'need to know' principle, not in terms of the therapist keeping back information which the client is deemed unable to handle, but in terms of the information being seen as relevant and useful by the client.

2. Present the information

Again the step is taken with awareness of the client's existing understanding. It is demanding of the therapist in that information needs to be couched in terms which are accessible to the client. The jargon of 'diagnosis', 'prognosis' and so on may benefit communication between professionals but can serve to promote an expert role for the therapist when used with clients.

3. Check the result

This is a return to listening: listening to reflections from the client. It is not to check whether the client has got the facts right, as the therapist sees them, but listening to the client's understanding of the information given and his responses in thought and feelings.

4. Ensure retention

The giving of information is a two-way process. It is not a one-off statement made by the therapist. It may be necessary for the therapist to repeat or restate the information in the light of responses from the client. It may be, too, that other forms of communication can help: in writing, pamphlets or even taping the conversation between the therapist and the client.

The usual way of thinking about providing information is to see it, as Davis (1993) does, as being information provided by the professional for the client. Clients can, however, also be a source of information for the therapist. An obvious example is parents who can provide therapists with detailed information about their particular child which is unavailable from any other source. Furthermore, some clients can have delved into and read about a medical condition and have more knowledge in a specific area than the therapist.

Client's concerns

There are two common experiences for people using counselling skills. The first is that clients often seem initially to talk about a particular experience, for instance, rather than what may be the real concerns. Similarly clients, in talking about their particular problems and possible solutions, can go off at a tangent and talk about many things which, on the surface at least, seem irrelevant. Though such behaviours can feel time wasting for the therapist, they can play an important role for the client in establishing and maintaining relationships. Talking about the weather, for instance, can be a way of relaxing, sharing mutual experiences and establishing trust. Nevertheless, though it is clearly important to follow the client's path, the therapist can help in clarifying what the path is. The second experience for helpers is that clients can talk in global terms about, for instance, being in pain, or feeling useless, or feeling down. These are, of course, important statements, but give the therapist no more than a general impression.

Challenging which focuses on the client's concerns, then, helps the client to clarify his path and to recognize specific signposts. Two processes are generally recognized: summarizing and concreteness. Summative reflections were discussed in Chapter 7. They can be, to use the words of Davis (1993: 85): 'gently challenging in that they may stimulate insight, understanding and a change in perspective.'

Summative reflection is a simple form of challenging in that there is little attempt to 'read between the lines' and feeds back to clients what they actually said, albeit in the therapist's own words. It is challenging to the degree that it is selective. Summative reflection can be challenging in that the therapist is summarizing what he sees as the client's most significant thoughts or feelings in tackling his concerns, and by omission is saying that other things the client has talked about are not so important. This is challenging through helping the client review his priorities and main concerns. When summative reflections are challenging they say to the client: you have talked about many important things, but these are the main concerns with which we should go forward. Such statements start with a phrase like, 'What we have talked about so far is . . . '.

Another process of focusing is often called 'concreteness'. This involves challenging clients to convey more precisely the meaning of the situation to them and their reactions to it. It is helping the client to talk about specific examples, instances or experiences and to go into specific details. Concreteness does not require a series of specific questions such as 'Where was the pain?', 'When did you have the pain?', 'How long did it last?' and so on, that is, questions preset by information that therapists think they should seek. It involves the therapist asking questions such as:

- 'what do you mean by . . . ?'
- 'when you say you feel . . . can you be more specific about exactly how you were feeling . . . ?'
- 'can you give me an example of when you felt . . . ?'

Concreteness, then, involves helping the client be more specific but does not necessarily involve asking specific closed questions.

Relationships and communication

Therapists are frequently challenged by their relationships and the processes of communication with clients. Challenges which centre on the immediate situation of helping, that is, the relationship between the therapist and the client, the process of helping, and aspects of the two-way flow of therapist–client communication, are sometimes called 'immediacy'. Perhaps the first thing to say about immediacy is that it is potentially very threatening. This is evident if we think of any relationship we have: to start to analyse honestly the relationship and the feelings involved requires a real strength of trust and genuineness from which questioning can begin, particularly if the questioning has negative connotations.

The process of helping is a meeting with 'self' as much as with the 'other', for both the provider and receiver of help. To engage in what Egan (1977) calls 'you–me talk', focuses attention not only on the relationship and communication between the therapist and the client but, directly or by implication, also on other relationships. We return, then, to the discussions in Chapter 1, where it was suggested that therapist–client relationships are understood in comparison to and in contrast with other relationships.

The following example is taken from a conversation between an occupational therapist (OT) and an elderly client who had just begun to use a wheelchair following an accident in his own home. They were exploring the various adaptations which would be required within the house if the client was to continue living in his own home as he wished. The therapist felt he had a good rapport with the client, but they might have been skating over some of the difficulties the client was experiencing.

OT   'We seem to be going like a train.'
Client   'Sorry?'
OT   'I mean we seem to be galloping along again. Perhaps we need to take things a little more slowly.'
Client   'That's my way. I like to get things done. I'm never one for too much chat.'
OT   'Yes, that's fine, but I was wanting to make sure that we get it right. Making sure it's how you want it. It's been a traumatic time for you.'
Client   'Don't worry about that. I'll keep you right.'
OT   'I suppose it's me too. I don't like rushing things. I like to make sure we've discussed all the possibilities. But it must be difficult for you, having had such an active life.'
Client   'Yes it's frustrating, but I can still be active can't I when we've made a few changes. But perhaps you're right. I'm always wanting to get down to business. Let's take stock.'

Immediacy can be helpful in a number of ways and there are elements of each in this exchange between the occupational therapist and his elderly client. It can:

- enhance the relationship between the therapist and the client
- help the client develop self-awareness in understanding his experiences, feelings and relationships with others
- help the therapist develop self-awareness in reflecting on his relationship and communication with the specific client, and clients generally.

Personal reflections 8.1

Think of times you have been challenged to re-evaluate your thinking and feelings. Think first of your relationships and experiences with clients. Can you specify examples of when you have been challenged by clients? Think too of your relationships generally. All the forms of challenging discussed in this chapter are part and parcel of our everyday relationships and communication, not just techniques which can facilitate the helping process in therapy.

Client's self-awareness

Challenges which focus on the client's developing self-awareness are an extension of the process of listening as conveyed by the Chinese symbol (Figure 7.1). It is essentially a process of reflecting the messages from the client, but demands of the client by drawing attention to or clarifying thoughts, feelings and meaning of which the client is either unaware or only partially aware. The general response that the therapist is seeking from the client is: 'Yes that's what I'm saying, but I had not seen it like that before.' Challenging of this type can take many forms, but we shall concentrate here on reflection and confrontation.

The dangers of challenging through reflection and confrontation are immediately apparent. They are complex, subtle processes which can have dramatic and far-reaching implications and consequences for the therapist–client relationship. Challenging through reflection can imply 'I know better than you do what you are thinking and feeling', while challenging through confrontation can have the more simple connotation, 'I think you are wrong.' Yet both can be deeply effective in helping the other person explore his concerns. We shall look first at reflection, building on the discussions in the previous chapter.

Reflecting feeling becomes challenging when the therapist is interpreting things the client has said or his non-verbal behaviour to suggest to the client he has feelings about his experiences which he is not explicitly expressing and of which he is perhaps not consciously aware, for instance, 'I'm getting the feeling that you are feeling guilty because you are not doing as much around the house as you used to and you feel this is unfair on others.' Expressing feelings can be threatening and sometimes inappropriate when they cannot be handled by either the client or the therapist. Nevertheless, established relationships in which there is a high degree of genuineness, acceptance and empathy can provide a context of trust and safety and a space in which feelings can be explored. Drauker (1992) provides a list of different ways in which this can be facilitated, one of which is reflecting feelings as mentioned above. A second is 'concreteness', that is, asking the client to specify and describe feelings associated with a particular experience. A third strategy is to suggest that others in the client's life may have certain feelings about what is happening, such as anger, sadness or pleasure, and ask whether the client is experiencing similar emotions. This has the danger of telling the client how he should be feeling. Drauker's fourth suggestion is a form of 'immediacy', as it involves discussing the difficulties of expressing emotions with the client.

Reflecting meaning, or 'advanced empathy', as discussed in Chapter 7, can take the form of 'You feel . . . because . . .' statments, which make links, that the client may be unaware of, between his emotions and his experiences or thoughts. Some books provide exercises involving lists of possible situations, and the reader is required to suggest possible responses which reflect meaning (Gazda *et al.*, 1977). Whether or not such exercises are useful, they are superficial in realizing the powerfulness of advanced empathy. Russell calls empathy 'the basic connective energy of human life'. She writes (1992: 11): 'To touch is to empathise, is to feel for, is to reach, is to connect. It is through this meaningful communication between two human beings that the energy for constructive change is transmitted.' In this light, pencil and paper exercises have very limited value. Challenging through reflecting meaning, or advanced empathy, is not a technique, but a resonance of intimacy and sensitivity between two people who have established harmony.

Davis provides a couple of examples:

'Perhaps you're getting upset with your son, when actually you are angry about your own inability to help him' is an example of this skill, addressed to a father who could not enjoy interacting with his son who had arthritis. Another example of advanced empathy is the following statement made to a mother who was trying to decide how to stop her son (with mild hemiplegia) from playing football, his passion, before he was dropped from the team. Although the mother had only talked about the child, the teacher said, 'But what is really upsetting is your own feeling of being unable to protect him any longer'. (1993: 87)

Davis goes on to say that in both cases the parents immediately began to weep and then went on to talk in length about their feelings and the reasons why they felt as they did. The examples show the possible power of advanced empathy, but they also illustrate the dangers. Unless the statements reflecting meaning are grounded in good listening and a strong relationship, the helper's suggestions might be rejected, simply upsetting or even downright insulting.

We turn next to the notion of confrontation, which as the term itself suggests is the most direct way to challenge a client, and certainly highlights the need for the context of challenging described above. When used to facilitate and support the exploration of the client's views and feelings it is not aggressive or combative as the common usage of the word implies. It involves pointing out discrepancies which emerge as the client explores his thoughts and feelings. These discrepancies can take a number of different forms:

1. Inconsistencies in what the client is actually saying.
2. Inconsistencies between verbal and non-verbal messages, say for instance:
   (a) The client says he is not in pain but all the non-verbal signs – eyes, posture, tone of voice and so on – contradict this.
   (b) The client describes intolerable pain, yet moves freely.
3. Differences between the client's self-image and ideal self.
4. Difference between how the client thinks and feels and what he actually does.
5. Differences between the client's and the therapist's understanding and feelings.

In the first instance, extreme care must be taken as messages, particularly non-verbal messages, are so difficult to interpret. The therapist might, for instance, misjudge the intensity of pain suffered by a client. Clients can hide or deny, even to themselves, the pain they are experiencing. Challenging the client in such circumstances may detract from the relationship and two-way flow of communication between him and the therapist, rather than helping him in self-exploration.

Confrontation by pointing out discrepancies demands considerable sensitivity and care on the part of the helper if it is to be effective in furthering the process of help and not destructive. It becomes even more problematic in the context of providing therapy in those situations in which the confrontation seems to be initiated by the therapist and reflects the therapist's concerns and agendas. A comprehensive list of all such difficult situations a therapist might face would be extensive and include circumstances in which:

- the therapist is 'breaking bad news' to the client
- the client is consistently negative, even abusive, towards the therapist or the process of therapy
- the client makes sexual innuendos and advances toward the therapist
- the therapist suspects that the client is either being abused or abusing others

- the client is repeatedly non-co-operative in therapy, having ostensibly agreed courses of action which are then not carried out, perhaps with a series of excuses for non-co-operation
- the client is consistently negative about himself ('I'll never be able to do that,' 'I'll try but it will be the same old story,' and so on) or negative about others in his life.

It has to be said, too, that this list only looks from the perspective of the therapist. A similar list might be drawn up of difficult situations clients can face in therapy.

Personal reflections 8.2

Above is a list of difficult, seemingly confrontational, situations that therapists can face.

1. Think of specific examples of these types of situations from your own experiences as a therapist. Can you think of difficult situations which are not covered in this list?
2. Write a description of each of these situations covering the following:
   (a) the particular circumstances and events
   (b) your views and feelings about the situation, including your thoughts about how you wanted the situation to change
   (c) repeat (b), but this time put yourself in the other person's shoes and try to answer from his viewpoint.
3. How has the situation been resolved, if it has? How might you have tackled it differently?

The nature of human relationships in helping is not such that a set of rules can be formulated which could apply to all such situations. Nevertheless, there are guidelines which are consistent with the principles outlined in Chapter 4 and the processes of relationships in Chapter 5:

1. Therapists may face situations in which they feel there is no alternative other than direct confrontation. Such direct

actions are best led by 'I' statements (Nelson-Jones, 1986), such as 'I feel . . .', 'I think . . .' and so on, rather than 'You' statements, such as 'You have . . .', 'You are . . .' and so on, which are blaming and more directly aggressive. The therapist should also, maybe against his inclinations, listen to the client's viewpoint.

2. Confrontation can sometimes be the most obvious action, but should always be thought about in relation to other possible ways of challenging, such as immediacy or self-disclosure. Referral can be a more positive option in some situations. The most obvious option in the human relations of helping is not always the best.

3. The therapist might seek support of various kinds, such as through discussion with a colleague who can act as a critical friend. While this can help, it can sometimes exacerbate the problem when support is unhelpful. I am thinking here of a therapist who approached his line manager, did not receive an empathetic or even sympathetic response, and felt even more isolated in the situation he faced.

4. All confrontations, however difficult the situation may be, should be approached with respect for the client and be directed towards a positive outcome which allows for disagreements and differences of opinion and can enhance the relationship between the therapist and the client.

Therapist's self-awareness

The process of developing the therapist's self-awareness is crucial to the use of counselling skills. It arises in the context of challenging, as demands for rethinking and re-evaluation are brought to bear on the therapist in his journey of exploration with the client. Again this can take many forms and emerge in different ways throughout the whole process of therapy, but we shall concentrate on what is often called 'self-disclosure'.

Self-disclosure was one of the bricks in the wall of not listening. There are, as Segal has recognized, many reasons for counsellors not to disclose information about themselves.

Segal's list includes the following (1993: 14): '. . . it is important for the counsellor to retain privacy and clear boundaries in
the relationship in order to be free to use their empathy to the
full in the service of the client.' However, regardless of
whether this is true in counselling, it seems to be questionable
when applied to the use of counselling skills by therapists in
the course of their work. The use of counselling skills is aimed
at breaking down rather than building up the 'clear boundaries
in the relationship'.

A very different idea of self-disclosure is presented by
Tschudin for whom it is a process of 'self-sharing'. She writes:

> Self-sharing can be tremendously liberating. Suddenly you feel
> equals, two human beings with each other, but the aim of self-
> sharing is not that *you* feel better, but that your client can move
> forward and perhaps feel less isolated. (1991: 89)

As self-sharing, self-disclosure is not simply a challenging
skill, it is integral to the whole use of counselling skills by
therapists, and we can return to the general points we made
earlier about challenging:

1. Self-sharing is part of the whole process of building the
   relationship and two-way communication. Statements
   which begin with phrases such as, 'I was once in a similar
   situation . . .' or 'I felt like that when . . .' are ways of being
   with the other person: a mutual sharing of feelings and
   experiences.
2. Self-sharing can build on listening and be part of attending,
   following and reflecting. Effective self-sharing continues
   down the path taken by the client. The aim is to allow
   clients to continue talking about their concerns as they
   see them. It is also part of the process of reflection in
   that therapists can monitor the client's reactions to the feelings and experiences he expresses in self-disclosing. Self-
   disclosure which is not grounded in empathy can be met
   with, 'No, it was not like that for me', or silence, or questions and discussion around the therapist's concerns rather
   than the client's.
3. Self-disclosure can be challenging when it helps the client
   to review personal experiences and feelings. It is effective

when the client continues exploring his personal concerns by using and building on what the therapist has said.
4. The central danger of challenging is the message to the client that therapists think they have 'heard this all before', and thus self-disclosure builds rather than demolishes the brick wall.

An example of self-disclosure comes from the work of a speech and language therapist (ST) and, in particular, a conversation with the mother of a young person with a severe articulation difficulty (George). The speech and language therapist had been working for some time with the family and had seen George at school. During this particular conversation George's mother had been saying that she hoped he was well accepted at school but was obviously worried by the fact he talked little about school.

> ST 'Listening to you reminds me of the problems I had with our Robert at school. He kept things to himself and it was ages before we found out he was being bullied by one of the older boys. It wasn't serious but I wish I'd found out sooner and got it sorted out.'

This challenge helped George's mother to see that, in a general sense, the difficulties she was experiencing with George at school were shared by other parents. It helped her to talk through her worries about George and discuss ways in which her concerns might be tackled.

Personal reflections 8.3

1. You should now look at your own practice in terms of the strategies you use for challenging clients. Use Table 8.1 to review and reflect on incidents, events and interactions that you have recorded in relation to the focuses of challenges and how you helped clients in re-evaluating their thinking feelings and actions.
2. Though role-play exercises can be successful, it is not easy to set up a situation in which you can practise skills of challenging. This is because of the strength of relationship required and the groundwork of listening.

Nevertheless, it is possible to repeat an exercise you have already used and this time concentrate on the challenging involved. It requires working with a partner again.

(a) The speaker should think of an unresolved problem in his life. Apply the stages of the counselling process in helping your partner work through this concern:

- defining the problem
- re-evaluating the problem
- his aims and goals in solving the problem
- an assessment of the relevant opportunities and personal resources
- an action plan of what the speaker proposes to do
- how he intends to evaluate the results of his efforts.

(b) The listener should reflect back to the speaker everything he has 'heard', including the responses to non-verbal as well as verbal messages.

(c) The speaker should reflect back to the listener what the experience of being listened to was like. The sort of questions that can be covered are:

- was the speaker able to share experiences, feelings and understandings?
- how well did the listener attend?
- what were the listener's thoughts, feelings and sensations throughout?
- at what points was the listener genuine, showing warmth or showing empathy?

(d) This particular exercise concentrates on the strategies of challenging used (Table 8.1). It is important for the person who has been doing the speaking to reflect back to the helper the points at which he felt he was being challenged and the points at which he felt he might have been usefully challenged. The listener should also report on his thoughts and feelings about challenging in this particular situation. How comfortable did you feel challenging someone

else? Were there points at which you felt you challenged and you should not have? Were there points
at which you might have been more challenging?

Questions which challenge

A specific context for challenging in the work of therapists is
the clinical interview. We shall concentrate here on a mainstay
of clinical interviewing: questioning. Questioning is in essence
challenging on the straightforward basis of demanding
answers. It can constitute an extreme form of challenging, as
in an interrogation: 'We have ways of making you talk!' One is
reminded of a stereotypical interrogation in which a light is
shone in someone's face and question after question is fired in
the person's direction. It is an extreme picture, maybe, but
looking at the lists of information that therapists can be
advised to gather in 'assessing the client's needs', an interrogation does not seem so far from what is required.

This is not to say that questioning is not a legitimate and
useful part of clinical interviewing, from both sides. It can be a
part of listening, as discussed in the previous chapter. It can
also play a valuable role in all the forms of challenging discussed above. Questioning can be part of a two-way flow of
communication, particularly if we take into consideration the
client questioning the therapist as well as the therapist doing
the questioning, as is more usual.

How, then, can questioning contribute to challenging and
enabling clients to rethink and re-evaluate their understanding, feelings and actions? The first requirement is that questioning should be part of the listening process of attending,
following, reflecting and the CAP as discussed in the previous
chapter. Questioning can then further each focus for challenging. Within each of the following is included an example
taken from the interviews between Edna and Katie, whose
circumstances were described in the Introduction.

Information

Questions have a role to play at each stage of providing information, from exploring the client's present understanding to reviewing the client's developing understanding when new information has been provided. At one point, for instance, Katie asked the seemingly straightforward question, 'What do you know about arthritis?' Edna answered by describing her own experiences, rather than in terms of the more general knowledge Katie wished to explore.

Client's concerns

Questions have an obvious role in eliciting specific examples of experiences, thoughts and feelings. A major concern for Edna, for instance, which slowly emerged during the interview, was her disappointment at having little contact with her son and his family. At one point Edna was talking about how she managed to travel to the hospital for appointments.

Edna   'Henry used to come through to take me, but he's been too busy lately.'

Katie   'It was useful getting lifts from your son.'

Edna   'Well it was a chance to see him and to catch up on all the news. But I can get a taxi.'

Katie   'So you don't see your son so much now. How do you feel about that?'

This question arose from Katie's feelings that Edna was touching on concerns which were important to her and her inclinations proved correct. The practicalities of travelling to and from the hospital which Edna repeatedly raised were minor compared to her feelings of isolation from her son and his family.

Relationships and communication

Questions can be used to focus on the immediate situation of the relationship and communication between the therapist and the client. A good example came from Edna rather than the therapist. During the third session she asked Katie, 'Do you like coming here to see me?' This question was more significant than it might have seemed. It reflected her lack of confidence in making new relationships which, though she never used these actual words, could be characterized as, 'Who would be interested in an old woman like me?', and seemed to be seeking affirmation that Katie was interested in her as a person rather than just 'doing her job'.

Client's self-awareness

As described above, this usually entails reflective statements rather than questions. Questions do have a part to play, for instance, in asking for feedback. During one of their later sessions, Katie was able to use the empathy that had developed with Edna to suggest, 'I think you are worried about getting in touch with Henry because you think he'll feel you are pestering him and what you really want is for it to come from him.' She then asked, 'Do you think I'm right?'

Therapist's self-awareness

Again this mainly involves statements which describe the therapist's experiences and feelings, but again questions can prompt responses. Staying with the explorations of Edna's relationship with her son to illustrate this, Katie said, 'I feel guilty sometimes myself about wanting to do a job and being there for the kids. They're getting old enough now but I wouldn't want them to think I wouldn't drop everything if they needed me. Do you think that Henry feels the same?' Katie was challenging Edna to recognize the possibility that she might be making assumptions about how her son was feeling.

Challenging questions

This is, intentionally, an ambiguous phrase. It captures the complexities of two-way flow. 'Challenging questions' can refer to demands made by the therapist in helping the client to reflect on experiences, feelings and actions. It can refer, too, to similar demands on the therapist by clients asking searching questions. It can also refer to processes of awareness and reflection on the part of the therapist and the client in reviewing the questions they ask in terms of immediacy, that is, the communication and relationship between the therapist and the client. This is standing back from and reviewing questions: a questioning of questions. The reviewing process is clearly evident in the following quote from a piece written by a woman with ME:

> I like the doctor's voice. He introduces himself, asks a few questions. Suddenly he says, 'Do you always wear makeup?' I feel exposed, vulnerable, and rage boils up inside me. I shout at him, 'How dare you ask such a question? Are you judging me by the way I look? What do you know of my life?' He stares at me in horror and walks out of the ward. Well, I might as well go home. I feel stricken, incredibly upset. Suddenly he is there in front of me again. 'Forgive me,' he says, 'I didn't mean to hurt you.' So I stay. (Sullivan, 1994: 95 – 96)

A distinction is often made between open and closed questions. Closed questions demand specific information usually requiring 'yes/no' or other one word answers: 'Can you cope in this situation?', 'How often does this happen?', 'Who helps when you have this problem?' Such questions have a number of connotations. Perhaps the first is that they demand information which can be 'right' or 'wrong'. Answers can be judged on a factual basis, such as responses to the question 'Do you feel pain when . . . ?'. They can also be judged on a value basis. This is easiest to see in questions such as 'Who do you live with?' with the possibility of, for instance, prejudice against single parent families. This can also, however, be inherent in questions such as 'How many children do you have?' or 'How often do you get out each week?' A second connotation is that the questioning is following the agenda or path of the therapist rather than that of the client. Closed questions can have the feeling of being concerned with the information the therapist thinks is required for his purposes rather than the client's concerns. It is for these reasons that closed questions can feel part of an interrogation: the information is required by the therapist and the client has to respond as well as he can.

Open questions seem less challenging in the sense that they are 'open' and leave space for the client to go down his own path, but they can be at least as personally challenging and threatening for clients. For instance, to ask 'Why?' questions is to question the person's feelings, understanding or actions on a personal basis. 'Why' questions can have an 'explain yourself' connotation. Open questions can also have a feeling of prying, demanding personal information. This connotation of open questions again raises issues which have been one of our recurring themes, that is the professionalizing and, more specifically medicalizing, of essentially private concerns. Open questions can instigate interventions into the values, feelings and personal life of clients. Thus, whereas closed questioning can be reflected on in terms of interrogation and all that this means for communication and relationships, open questions can be reflected on in terms of the, perhaps subtle, manipulation of the client by the therapist and all that this means for the process of communication and relationships. The words 'interrogation' and 'manipulation' may seem very negative but do not necessarily suggest Machiavellian motives on the part of the therapist. Questioning is integral to the flow of communication and defines the therapist–client relationship and should be the subject of reflection by the therapist in terms of the human relations of therapy.

There are a number of ways in which therapists can review their questioning of clients. The first is in terms of their own and the client's understanding of the questions being asked. For instance, multiple questions, that is, questions requiring two or more answers, can be confusing for both the client and the therapist; for example, 'Do you experience pain and need help in dressing?' Vague questions can be equally difficult to answer and the responses difficult to understand; for example, 'Can you cope with household chores?' A third example is the use of jargon in questions. As French says, specifically in relation to physiotherapy:

> Every profession and occupation has its jargon and the physio-
> therapy profession is certainly no exception. It is a common

mistake to use medical terms and jargon when questioning or communicating information to patients. (1992: 158)

She goes on to say, however, that it is important not to be patronizing. In the context of our present discussions, it is also important to emphasize the need for therapists to reflect on their use of jargon and the responses, embarrassment, clarity of understanding and so on, in clients' responses.

A second way of reviewing questions is in terms of the way in which the actual question itself shapes and influences the client's responses. Leading questions contain assumptions which may not be challenged by the client. The question 'How often do you feel pain?' presumes the client feels pain. The question, 'How often do strangers misunderstand what you are saying?' presumes there are situations in which the client is not understood. Again, French (1992) adds a caveat. She suggests that leading questions can convey to the client that experiences, feelings and actions are to be expected and are acceptable. Thus, to ask how often a person takes time off work because of backache suggests that this is an understandable possibility. It can also be argued that a leading questions is not really a type of question at all, but being leading is a quality of all questions. The questioning of questions, then, needs to focus on the degree to which the questioning follows the client's path of understanding and thinking. Thus, the question 'How often do you feel pain?' is leading if it comes from the therapist's predetermined agenda of important questions to ask. It is less leading if the client is already talking about his concerns about frequently being in pain.

A third way of looking at questions has already been mentioned above, that is, in terms of their value-basis. The question itself can be loaded with values about how the client should or ought to think, feel or act. Again this is often seen as a category of questions: 'loaded' or 'value-laden'. An example given by Burnard (1989) is, 'Have you stopped beating your wife?' It can be argued, however, that all questions can be value-laden, even if just on the basis of suggesting that certain information is of importance. Even questions such as, 'Who do you live with?' suggest that this is significant information and holds the possibility of value-judgements about responses, for example, if the client is living with a partner of the same sex. Again, then, the value-basis of questions provides important grounds for reflection.

Finally, given the challenging nature of questioning, it is important for the therapist to remember that direct questions are not the only technique for gathering information or exploring understanding and feelings. Macchielli summarizes the problem succinctly:

> He (doctor or therapist) is in danger of being carried away by the medical model: to get on as quickly as possible, ask numerous questions related to the hypotheses that arise after a first look at the problem, and give his diagnosis or his advice as soon as the case has fitted into one or other of his categories. (1983: 78)

He suggests a strategy which I have found to be useful, that is to conduct the interview by 'announcing the theme and then letting the client approach it and develop it as he wishes' (1983: 80). Thus, for instance, in taking a history relating to the particular problem presented, the therapist would approach the interview with a list of possible topics to be covered rather than a list of specific questions. Each topic covered could be introduced with a statement starting with a phrase such as, 'Tell me about . . .'. This is often referred to as semi-structured interviewing as opposed to a structured interview.

Personal reflections 8.4

1. If possible you should review an interview you have undertaken with a client: questioning the questions. This can be done from a transcript, but transcribing takes a lot of time and you can do this by listening to an audio tape you have made of the interview.

    (a) Make a note of as many as possible of the questions you asked. How many were open and how many were closed?

    (b) Do you think that you and the client had a shared understanding of the questions? Were some questions vague, confusing or difficult to understand in any way?

(c) Were any of the questions leading? Were you making assumptions in the way any of the questions were worded?

(d) Were the questions in any way value-laden or reflecting clear presumptions on your part? How do the questions reflect your beliefs and values?

(e) Were there any points at which the questions you asked were unnecessary and the information might have been gained by simply introducing the topic for discussion?

2. This is a point at which you could review your journal writing in general.

(a) Are you writing a sufficiently detailed description of incidents and so on for you to be able to reflect on yourself, your feelings, understandings and actions?

(b) How are you handling the questions of the time required in undertaking your journal writing? This has always been the greatest problem for students I have worked with.

(c) How is keeping a journal working for you? Make a list of the gains you have made from this activity.

(d) Have you shared your journal with anyone else? Might you become confident enough to do so? How are you handling issues of confidentiality?

(e) How might you tackle your journal a little differently as a vehicle for raising self-awareness?

Part Three

In Context

9

A Multi-professional Context

Too many cooks?

A comic scene which the idea of helping can conjure up is that of an old lady being dragged across a road by an over-enthusiastic boy scout. The scene becomes more like black comedy when a multi-professional team is envisaged helping a disabled child to eat a meal: a physiotherapist to ensure the child is sitting and holding her head in the correct position; an occupational therapist to advise on the design of the chair, cutlery and so on; a speech and language therapist to monitor the chewing of the food and movement of the tongue; a teacher taking the child through a self-help eating programme; a dietician to advise on nutritional value; and so on. A comic scene, maybe, but it is not such a fantasy when it is remembered that there are over 40 different types of professional who can be involved in helping disabled people.

It is not such a comic scene to the Willsons either, as parents of a young woman with profound and multiple impairments:

> One of the most difficult things in caring for Victoria is the number of people in her life. I counted them. In any one day, there could be twenty-seven people handling her! This includes the care staff who get her up, wash her and dress her. There's the escort and the bus driver who take her to school, the school cook and the dinner ladies, her teacher and three teaching assistants, and the school nurse. She comes back to tea with the afternoon shift, and goes to bed with the night staff. In addition she might see a doctor, visit the

hospital or have a dental appointment. She might see the physio-therapist, the occupational therapist or the speech therapist. There may be a special programme like swimming or horse riding, and the people involved in those activities. There are a lot of people involved in her little life! (Atkinson and Ward, 1986: 36)

Critiques of professionals have come from people who have looked at the whole 'professionalizing' of help in our society. What they say, essentially, is that a professionalized service creates dependency in that it takes away people's capacities to cope with and control their own lives. McKnight (1977) gives a detailed breakdown of what he calls the 'disabling effects' of professionalization of help. First there are assumptions of need:

1. Needs are socially constructed. Professionals focus on the individual, the client, and need is translated into a defi-ciency of the individual. It is an unfortunate absence, emp-tiness or lack in the person, rather than say a right, or a want or an obligation to others. Thus, Mcknight sum-marizes the message as: 'You are deficient.'
2. In this social construction of need, the perceived deficiency is *in* the client. There is something wrong with the indi-vidual. The message is: 'You are the problem.'
3. As systems of techniques and technology have advanced, professionals' work has become increasingly specialized. The person is chopped into pieces with an expert to cater for each problem, each need, as in the multi-profes-sional team example suggested above. Thus the third message in these assumptions of need is: 'You have a collection of problems.'

There are, then, assumptions about remedy of need:

1. The message of the first of these assumptions is that: 'As you are the problem, I am the answer.' You, the client, are not the answer; nor are your family or friends; nor is the social and economic environment. Professionals are the experts and have the answers. It is also assumed, of course, that problems can be solved.

2. As techniques and technologies have advanced, professionals and their 'tools' have defined the needs of their clients to which they are the answer. Thus the remedy defines the need.

3. As experts with expertise which they are paid for, professionals have coded the problem and the solution into their own language, or jargon, which is incomprehensible to clients. If everyone had the expertise, who would pay professionals! So the message is: 'You are incapable of understanding your problem.'

4. Finally, as only professionals can know what the problem is and only they have the answers, or techniques, to solve the problem, only they can decide whether the help has been effective. The final message according to McKnight is then: 'You are unable to know whether you have been helped.'

In the final part of this book we look at this broader context of the human relations of helping through therapy, particularly in relation to questions of power and powerlessness. We are recognizing that turning principles into practice takes place in a context of existing relationships, expectations, roles and responsibilities. We are recognizing, too, that the book is about processes of helping involving decisions which affect people's lives.

This chapter is a case study of the views and concerns of different groups of people in a specific situation: a multi-professional context, including a doctor, a nurse, teachers, physiotherapists, a speech therapist, social workers and residential care workers. It is an examination of the say that young disabled people and their helpers have in decisions which shape their lives.

Ashdown School is a school for young disabled people from 3 to 19 years old. In the spring of 1991 a research project was used to further the discussions in drawing up the School Development Plan and in the Staff Development Programme. The research was undertaken by myself and Carole Thirlaway at the request of the school. As researchers we attended meetings of mixed groups of professionals and parents and conducted open-ended discussions/interviews with students, teachers, other professionals, parents and residential care workers, a total of 30 people. These discussions were based around a series of topics (see below) that we suggested after attending a number of preliminary meetings. As part of the research, a report was presented to the school based on what people had said to us. This report was then discussed at two further meetings of professionals and parents.

The following is a copy of a sheet that we used to explain the research to the participants at Ashdown:

In the education and lives of young disabled people many decisions are made about: schools attended; what is studied; future careers; home and family circumstances; leisure pursuits; relationships with peers and friends; and so on.

Many people can be involved and have a say in these decisions, including: young people themselves; parents; friends; teachers; doctors; other professionals; and so on.

Many factors may influence these decisions, including: legal requirements; access and opportunity; resources; money; and so on.

In this study we are interested in your views about:

- who has a say in the decisions which affect young people's lives and education
- what stops people having more control
- how people work together in making decisions.

We would like to emphasize that it is *your* views that matter. We shall not be making recommendations or even commenting on people's views. Our job in this study is to find out and report the views of everyone without bias.

You might like to discuss the following:

- the say you have in decisions which affect young disabled people's education and lives, and what limits the say you have
- the say others have
- the say young people themselves have
- the implications of 'disability' on the decision-making that determines young people's education and lives.

The project aimed to collect and report the different perceptions, interests and judgements of all the participants in relation to decision-making. We tried to emphasize that we did not aim to make judgements about the relative effectiveness, success or failure of the school or anyone at the school. The research was to find out what was happening and why, rather than measuring how well the school was doing. All the interviews were confidential and all the quotes are anonymous.

Questions of professional power

A major area of concern for the professionals was the co-ordination and organization of their work in developing a multi-professional or team approach. This included both collaboration in decision-making and planning, and the co-ordination of their daily work in helping young people and their families. We shall look first at this distribution of power between professionals, looking from the viewpoint of the professionals themselves, before bringing parents and the disabled young people into the picture.

For all the professionals involved, the creation of an effective multi-professional team was 'essential' and 'vital'. From all that was said, it was possible to begin to define what was meant by an 'effective multi-professional team'. Major factors were:

- agreed goals and priorities in the help being offered to young people to co-ordinate the work of all involved
- trust in personal and professional relationships
- open, full and regular communication between professionals, both in periodic formal meetings and in informal daily contacts
- parity and equality in decision-making, in that the views of all were heard, valued and taken into account.

The suggestions in this list will be familiar aims for many professionals. Nevertheless, the list has been compiled more from statements about what the professionals wanted to see happening than from their descriptions of what they believed actually was happening. The overwhelming view was that such a multi-professional approach was not being achieved at Ashdown School. For some professionals it was not effective for some young people and for other professionals it was ineffective in some particular respects, but for all involved these issues were crucial to them in their work. The following are some examples of general doubts raised:

> That's a very fundamental issue that we haven't confronted. We just believe that it's better to work together in a multi-disciplinary team, but I'm not actually sure: (a) whether it is possible; and (b) that we are actually helping anyone by doing so. (Doctor and Sister)

A major problem pointed to was simply that there was not enough time in the day for all the professionals to provide all the help they saw as being necessary:

> Everyone wants to do their best and there isn't space to get that in. (Physiotherapists)

> If a child needs to be on its feet and needs to have therapy then I can see that the physiotherapists feel that that's of most importance, but it's frustrating to all of us when there is such a limited amount of time. (Teachers)

Hence there was a perceived need for agreed priorities. The basis for such collaboration was seen to lie within effective relationships and two-way communication between professionals. Relationships, however, tended to be seen as basically problematic:

> It's difficult sometimes, particularly if you don't agree with what they're suggesting. There's a certain amount of trust that has to come in here and if you think someone will always say that their role or need is greater than yours, well I'm afraid that's quite hard to accept. (Teacher)

The main difficulty seemed to be that while the professionals thought they put a lot of time and energy into communicating with each other, there were too many failures and breakdowns in communication. For instance, a group of professionals met weekly at what was called the 'communication meeting', but they felt it to be 'communication' in name only:

We have a meeting at 1 o'clock every Tuesday, which is multi-professional . . . we weren't sure we were communicating. Although we might have been giving information, whether anything was being done with the information, whether it was two-way or multi-way communication, we were concerned. (Doctor and Sister)

Finally, the crucial issue for the professionals involved was one of equality in terms of the balance of power between them in the decision-making process about the lives and education of young disabled people. The professionals sought a system in which they could have a say, that is, have their views listened to and taken into account. In terms of our present discussion, professionals sought power and raised their voices against what they saw as their own disempowerment. This was expressed in many ways:

I think we've both felt quite recently that we're finding it very difficult to give another contribution, because we've contributed so much in the past with what would seem so little result. (Doctor and Sister)

In a set-up like this, no one has the right to make arbitrary decisions about children. (Physiotherapists)

. . . this business about decision-making and just paying lip-service to the idea that we all can contribute, and I just don't think that happens . . . (Social Workers)

This struggle for power was seen by some as being within a particular social and historical context. For instance, both the teachers and the medical personnel felt that there had been a shift in recent years from medical to educational dominance in decision-making. The whole process of working together and decision-making had been 'de-medicalized' and educational priorities had taken precedence.

To summarize, these questions of professional power can be looked at in many ways, but what emerged for us was that the system itself had become the problem for professionals. It creates its own needs which have become major concerns for professionals and to which much time, energy and resources are devoted. Questions of professional power are essentially power struggles which are fought out and rationalized on the basis of professionals' perceptions of young people's needs.

Questions of parental power

Where do parents fit into the equations? Looking to the different viewpoints expressed in the research, the first answer to this question must be: it depends whose point of view you take. The differences between parents themselves and also between professionals was such that it was difficult to encapsulate the 'parental viewpoint' or 'the professional viewpoint' where questions of power relations between the two groups were concerned. Nevertheless, there were some consistencies in the patterns of differences between the two groups which seemed to indicate some fundamental conflicts and power struggles. In more general terms, such differences are expressions of the relations between a formal system and informal networks of people providing help.

Looking from the point of view of the professionals first, there was a widely recognized need to involve parents in their work and to take the parents' views into account in decision-making about their children. The research, for instance, originated from an initiative by teachers to strengthen what they called 'parental involvement' in the school. The following quote is indicative of the professionals' position:

> I feel the mums have felt quite important. I know some of them, you can pinpoint a few of them, who you can see have actually blossomed by having something, by feeling important and feeling as if they've contributed to what we're doing. (Teacher)

At the same time it was also recognized that parents tended to lack power within Ashdown:

> I think parents are often faced with panels of professionals advising them. I think in a case like that you have to be quite a strong and articulate parent to argue against professional decisions or ask for alternatives. (Teacher)

It seemed that the relationship professionals sought with parents was in some ways similar to the relationship they sought with other professionals, particularly in terms of agreed goals and priorities, and trust. There were many indications, however, that equality was only sought on professionals' terms and the involvement of parents was seen as a means of furthering the work of professionals. Thus, for instance, the physiotherapists argued that parents should have a say in decisions but only when they understood the consequences of those decisions as seen by the physiotherapists:

> To say to the family, if you're not going to be able to co-operate with that (i.e. the advice of professionals) or don't feel that that's important, what do you feel is important? Do you feel schooling is more important than what they are doing physically? Spell out to them the consequences of their choice . . ., but put the decision with them.'

> Routines need the co-operation and agreement of parents, . . . so there is a discussion of what will happen if a particular line is not taken . . . deterioration of the condition.

The doctor and sister simply said that they, 'work for parents having a different understanding'.

The relationship that professionals saw themselves as having with parents was directly associated with perceptions of their own power to influence decisions, though this emerged in different ways. To the extent that professionals lacked influence, or thought they lacked influence, over parents they felt themselves disempowered. The heart of the matter is that the 'need for parental involvement' is the professionals' need to ensure that parents share their view of what is required in the child's life and education. Professionals can see themselves as able to speak on behalf of their clients. For instance, the doctor and sister felt that they had built up trust with the parents they worked with by always consulting and informing them about their work with their child, and so in communication with other professionals they: 'want to be listened to representing the child's needs or parents' needs'.

Let us turn now to look at the views and experiences of the parents themselves. The research suggested first of all that theirs was a very different viewpoint. Though the parents themselves differed quite radically in the opinions and beliefs expressed, the pattern that emerged was considerably different to the professional point of view. For parents, involvement at Ashdown did not mean a say in decision-making within the school, but rather help for them in the sense that they 'want a break' and they were 'only too pleased to see them go off to school'. One parent in a conversation about whether parents had any influence in the running of the school stated:

> I think that would probably be the case with most parents, they just put their kids out to school in the morning. . . . In general most parents just let the school run itself without having much say about what goes on until they need to come to school.

They could find even the most basic contact with the school a traumatic experience. As one parent said: 'It's an amazing experience coming through the school gates. Your heart sinks. You know the teachers there are going to be ogres'. Furthermore, parents questioned whether the professionals at Ashdown really 'would want a lot of parental involvement'.

Thus parents saw the running of Ashdown and the help provided there as largely the responsibility of the professionals. Contact with the school tended to be thought of as happening when any problem arose with their particular child. Their satisfaction with the school was expressed in terms of whether they felt welcomed and listened to when such problems arose. Parents who felt they were listened to when problems arose with their child felt that they had a good relationship with Ashdown, or more usually one particular professional at the school. Others felt frustration and argued that they should be listened to as they had knowledge about and experiences with their child which the professionals could not possibly have. Ted's mother, talking of a particular disagreement with one member of staff, stated:

> I felt he was always saying, 'I'm right'. You didn't have an opinion. You couldn't give your opinion. His decision was right, full stop, you know . . . and they are telling me I'm wrong. But they only know Ted in Ashdown. They don't know what he's like outside, at home . . . I think the family or mother knows more.

Some parents, again particularly when their child was experiencing problems, simply wanted to know more about the child's life at Ashdown. This was not a call for more information, such as about the child's academic achievements or progress in therapy, but a wanting to know about the child's day-to-day life within the school. One parent stated, 'I'd like to be able to wander in like a fly on the wall'.

The parents also talked about a number of their major concerns which were not mentioned by the professionals. Many parents, for instance, expressed concerns about the family as a whole rather than just their son or daughter, including: their child waking at night and disturbing others' sleep; other children in the family wanting their friends to visit them at home; and the effect of 'emotional disturbance' in the home. One parent stated:

> I don't get up much to Ashdown school now, you know. With George being seventeen I sort of spend all my time with the little one now, because he's sort of had his childhood now. . . . I don't have much time actually because I work and then I come in and I've got to see to the kids and what have you.

Parents also talked about their child's lack of social life ('he just doesn't get out of the house'); associated with this were access barriers to local facilities ('they've just built a new Leisure Centre . . . but you can't get in with the wheelchair'); lack of access to public transport; and, as in the following quote, financial difficulties.

> Biggest problem is money. It's costing me more money now than it's ever done. It's the fares. It's gonna cost more than the mobility allowance and that's just the fares. He's never gonna get a chance to save up for a car or that, you know. (Parent)

A major point of discussion for the parents was their relationship with each other rather than the professionals at Ashdown. There was a Mothers' Support Group which met weekly in a room kept especially for the group at the school. Professionals could only attend this group when asked by the parents and they seemed to guard their independence with some jealousy. They seemed to find it a haven in a professionally dominated institution. For instance, they resisted any idea that parental involvement might be facilitated if meetings with professionals were to be held in their room.

They were also a group with their own identity and loyalties. The parents saw this group and other parents generally as a major source of help:

> We all have friends outside this group but you can't talk to any of them about your particular child's problem. I've lived in the village I live in for two years and there is very few people in that village even know I have a daughter, you know, because she's never out in the village life or whatever. (Parent)

The group also offered parents the opportunity to provide help:

> I went to help others with a handicapped kid. I've had problems all my life so I went to help. There was one woman there with a kid who was incontinent. . . . Martin was incontinent 'till about five and I used to say 'come on we'll pull the plug', and he thought it was great, you know (laughter). I helped her, maybe in a small way anyway. (Parent)

To summarize these questions of parental power, the heart of the parents' struggle with the professionals is in defining needs or problems. As a source of conflict this took on many forms. One particularly telling example came in a discussion during one of the joint meetings of the professionals and parents. The Head teacher introduced the question, 'who defines the problem' for discussion within the meeting, and at that point the discussion became dominated by professionals, until one of the parents spoke. She described how her son did not have friends in the local community because he did not attend the same school. He travelled some distance to Ashdown. She then rounded on the Head teacher and asked, 'Is that *your* problem?' The question was avoided by the Head teacher who gave a rationale for the existence of special schools, that is, scarcity of resources and professional input.

Again, then, 'the system' of professional support developed in our society creates the problem and the need. This is also one example of the contradictory position of professionals towards parents. In many ways they covertly undermined the very parental involvement they overtly intended. This defining of the problem seemed to us to be central in that professionals were putting parents in a position of non-involvement by predetermining the terms of involvement.

Questions of disabled people's power

Again let us look at this from the different points of view, starting with the professionals and then moving to the parents, and finally to disabled people themselves. For professionals, the issues raised are perhaps most simply seem as dilemmas. On one hand, from the professionals' viewpoint, young disabled people, needed their help if they were to become 'independent' and have control over their own lives. Without their help there would be deterioration, as most obviously stated by the physiotherapists:

> We've got some children in school with some horrendous leg deformities whose walking is very slow, very laboured and it – the walking – never happens anywhere else other than in school. So the actual independence of that person in terms of being able to stand is very limited. If they followed the regime like some of the other young people, they would be a lot more mobile and more well generally, because the implications of not doing some things affect not only the mobility but the actual kidney function, digestion and other things.

> Put a child in a wheelchair at an early stage and some lose the motivation to want to move themselves. It's easier to have somebody to push you . . . often round town they are being pushed and if you look at their faces they've switched off. The minute you push them it's like being driven in a car . . . if you sit as a passenger you haven't always taken notice of where you are going . . . I think that increases their disability.

Professionals also recognized that the very help provided can disempower young people, that is to say it can deny them of the very control over their lives and education it seeks to promote. This then is the heart of the dilemma for professionals: help is needed, but help can render young people more helpless. Such disempowerment is seen in two ways. First, the system is such that young disabled people are denied control by being passed from the hands of one professional to another in what seems at times to be a whirlwind of help. Let us return to the physiotherapists for some indicative statements: 'We then create pressures on the kids because we're rushing them'; 'It's like a sausage machine'; 'The children are wrapped up all the time'; and 'We make them more passive'.

Secondly, the actual processes of help were seen as disempowering in that decisions were being made about young people, their lives and education, by people who 'know best'. These can be seen as dilemmas which anyone who works with or helps young people in any way can face: how far should they be allowed, or encouraged, to take risks and learn for themselves and how far should they be guided by those who 'know best'? With young disabled people the questions become more extreme because their lives are filled with so many more people who 'know best', that is, professionals and parents, and who have power to control their lives. Furthermore their circumstances, such as lack of opportunities to truant, do not allow young people to rebel against the control of others. The doctor and sister summarized their way of working, for instance, as:

> . . . a fine balance between doing what's in the child's best interests for now and also considering the future. Sometimes there's an imposition on the child. . . . It's always a dilemma of how much do you impose what you feel is best.

Finally, we selected the following quote as a clear thought-provoking statement by a professional about the powerlessness of young disabled people and the role that professionals themselves play in the denial of power.

> I think they have very little say from the point of diagnosis to treatment or anything. They are made very dependent on a variety of specialists for information and advice . . . and in fact so are the parents. They're forced into a position of dependence and in fact how do you expect a disabled child to be independent when even their parents aren't? (Social worker)

Looking next from the parents' point of view, like the professionals they tended to see their child as disempowered, through being 'told what to do and not being given an explanation of why':

I honestly do not think my child is encouraged in any way, possibly because his life is short . . ., to take charge of his life and I think this might be giving him an unspoken message that you don't count.

When he's eighteen he's not a child any longer and he is entitled to his opinion and somehow I don't think they've got the time or the staff to cope with this.

Again, however, there were real differences between parents and professionals. For the parents, their starting point to considering questions of disabled people's power was by and large their child as a person. Parents saw themselves as relating to and helping their child, for instance, to overcome disability. In emphasizing this, parents would point to others as concerned with disability rather than the person. One parent at a meeting of the Mothers' Group had a lot of support when she stated, 'That's what's wrong with society as a whole: they don't see the person'. At a meeting of both professionals and parents the mother of a profoundly disabled young child stated that she had always wanted a professional to say something positive about her child that had nothing to do with problems. She found she was usually greeted with a positive statement, but about his perceived problems, for example, 'He's breathing better today'. What she wanted was a comment such as 'His hair's looking nice today', or 'I do like that jumper he's wearing'. Again, then, the parent was pointing to concerns about the child as a person rather than concentrating on impairment.

The young person's wishes and interests were used by parents to justify past decisions and decisions about the future. These were usually the young person's desires as understood by the parent, rather than the young person's needs as defined by professionals. Thus, for instance, one parent spoke of the decision that her son should attend courses at a local college as follows: 'I was at the school, but it was James's decision. It was up to him because he knew his own abilities. He knows better than I do, you know.'

Along similar lines, parents tended to talk about what they saw as their child's personal responses to the problems they faced – often emotional responses:

> It's so depressing at times . . . why, for instance, on Friday he
> came in at ten o'clock. I said, 'John is there something wrong'.
> He said, just out of the blue, 'I might as well not be here'. I said,
> 'What do you mean?' and he says, 'Well I'm always going to be
> there'. I says, 'oh don't talk like that John'.

John might have been talking about Ashdown school, but
his mother focused on John's emotional response. Parents saw
their children as having a lot to put up with, more than non-
disabled young people. Two main lines emerged in parents
thinking about the help they provided in this context. The first
was in helping their child to keep trying:

> I could cry for him when I see him, but you can't let him see
> how you feel. . . . I say you've got to help yourself. You've got
> to get off your backside. Just 'cos you've got a disability you
> can't just sit there. And I push him and push him, you know.

The second direction for help which parents spoke of was in
helping young people cope with their frustrations when they
thought they could not do things which they might want to,
such as playing football, a regularly quoted example.

> These children, they have natural feelings and they want to
> know why they can't do these things . . . and you're trying to
> explain why they can't do these things and help them to come
> to terms with disability within that age group.

We look next from the young disabled people's viewpoint at
these questions of disabled people's power. The research did
involve collecting and reporting the views of some students at
Ashdown. Though the time-scale involved prevented an in-
depth analysis of students' views, there were some indications
that students seek greater control of their lives in school, as in
the following couple of quotes:

> You are treated very much as a child even when you're sixteen,
> seventeen, eighteen year old. They say you're an adult but
> because you are still in the school situation you still get treated
> as a child.

> I think we should have more say, now that we're older.

One instance of collective action was discussed by a small
group of students:

'Except for the dinner queue, the dinner nannies always push to the front. The people in wheelchairs, it's fair enough that they can't get their own dinner, but they should at least go to the back of the queue like we have to, but they push straight to the front. There's not really much choice left by the time we get to the front of the queue.'

'And, like, we've complained about it but nothing's been done.'

'To whom have you complained?'

'We drew a petition up to the headmaster but he hasn't done anything yet.'

'So what do you think you'll do next?'

'Talk to someone else. Try to work something out.'

The involvement of the students in the whole school development programme was confined to these interviews. In policy-making meetings in which the School Development Plan was being reviewed, in staff development meetings at which student participation was debated, and in the Governors' meetings, the interests of students were represented by others. Furthermore, all the professionals at Ashdown were non-disabled, including the researchers, and no representative from local groups of disabled people has been consulted or invited to contribute to the school development programme in any capacity. This, then, is a central paradox which underpins the dilemmas facing professionals at Ashdown: the argument for the participation of disabled students in the decision-making processes which shaped their lives and education is largely pursued in the school by non-disabled professionals.

The questions of disabled people's power when looked at from the differing viewpoints of the various groups of participants at the school can be summarized as follows. As with questions of parental power, the key differences lie in defining needs or problems. However, we would suggest that with regard to questions of disabled people's power, this can best be understood in terms of differing viewpoints regarding the actual definition, or meaning, of 'disability'. Inherent within the views of participants are definitions of disability as:

- a 'personal tragedy' (Oliver, 1990) or problem inherent within the individual

- a system or administrative category
- the barriers faced in a world designed by and for non-disabled people.

Overall it could be argued that from the professionals' viewpoint, student participation in decision-making is seen either in personal tragedy terms, such as a need for decision-making skills, or in system terms, such as organizing multi-professional work. One crucial dimension of the question of disabled people's power is segregation, deriving from the fact that Ashdown School is a segregated provision in which young disabled people have been separated from their non-disabled peers. In terms of questions of disabled people's power, the first thing to be said is that, even in more recent statements in the literature relating to integration, no mention is made of young people themselves determining the process. They are the recipients, or not, of other people's decisions.

Questions of disabled people's power in relation to segregation, however, are more complex than simply a lack of say. It can be argued, for instance, that student participation in decision-making at Ashdown, particularly on the professionals' terms, can preserve status quo in segregation. There are a number of ways in which this can operate. At its most straightforward, segregation can be justified by the idea that young people, and their parents, have a say in the decision that they attend Ashdown, that is 'segregation by choice'. The second point we want to make in this context is perhaps less obvious. It can be argued that education at Ashdown School not only segregates young disabled people from their non-disabled peers, it also segregates them from disabled adults, in particular, the disability movement. Ultimately it has to be asked whether non-disabled professionals, not withstanding their good intentions, prepare young disabled people for life as disabled adults who are conscious of their identity as disabled people and of the struggle for full participative citizenship within our society. The struggle of voices (see Chapter 10), with regard to the definition of disability, is not about academic niceties, but about people's identities, lifestyle and quality of life.

In the final chapter we shall explore the possibilities of developing a reflective approach to human relations of helping in such multi-professional contexts.

Personal reflections 9.1

The personal reflection exercises for this chapter involve planning and undertaking a small-scale research project designed to further your development in the human relations of helping. Schön (1983: 68) writes: 'When someone reflects-in-action, he becomes a researcher in the practice context.'

The term 'researcher' can feel intimidating if it has all the connotations of knowledge and skills which you do not see yourself as possessing as a therapist. However, to the extent that you have engaged in the 'reflective practitioner' approach of this book and undertaken the exercises we have suggested in the 'Personal reflections', you are already in Schön's terms a researcher. Nevertheless, you will find it useful to read French (1993), who provides a practical account of the many research methods and approaches available to therapists. Here we shall provide only a very brief outline of the steps or stages in planning and undertaking a project (adapted from French, 1993, and Bell, 1987):

1. *Select a topic.* Perhaps the thinking and talking you have engaged in whilst reading this book and carrying out the 'Personal reflections' will have raised issues which you would like to explore in greater depth. It is important, however, to keep this small scale and manageable.
2. *Decide on the precise objectives and research question.* What exactly are you hoping to find out about in this project? You will need to be quite clear about this. It can be useful to explain the project to someone else at this stage.
3. *Plan the research.* A period of planning is essential. As mentioned in Chapter 1, the ethical issues in using counselling skills are similar to those in conducting research.

Securing the informed consent of everyone involved, for instance, is part of the planning of the research. This will require clarity about the aims of the research and what it will involve for yourself and others. How will you collect information or evidence? Observation, using videos for instance, and interviewing have already been discussed in previous chapters.

4. *Collect the information.* The key to this is to collect as careful and as full a record as possible: the notes you make, any documentation, audio tapes and so on.

5. *Analyse the data.* This, as French (1993) writes, is 'a major and exciting aspect of the research process'. Your approach to analysis can be more or less structured as discussed in relation to observation in Chapter 6.

6. *Write-up and dissemination.* Research can involve writing a formal report of the project and disseminating your findings to others. In the type of reflective practitioner exercise recommended here, in which the aim is self-development, this is important but need not be formal. It can again be part of your discussions with a partner or critical friend, and it can be particularly useful to discuss your findings with those who participated in your research, for instance someone you interviewed.

10

Reflecting in Context

Reflecting on reflections

> I am doing it
> the it I am doing is
> the I that is doing it
> the I that is doing it is
> the it I am doing
> it is doing the I that am doing it
> I am being done by the it I am doing
> it is doing it
> One is afraid of
> the self that is afraid of
> the self that is afraid of
> the self that is afraid
> One may perhaps speak of reflections
> (Laing, 1970: 84)

In this concluding chapter we shall be reflecting on the case study of the multi-professional context at Ashdown School. The research will provide a context for drawing together some of the main issues in the human relations of helping faced by therapists as reflective practitioners. First, however, we need to return to this whole idea of reflection and consider it in a little more detail. The notion of reflection or reflecting has recurred throughout the previous chapters, not least in the 'Personal Reflections'. In a restricted sense the notion of reflection refers to a form of teaching and learning which has been taken up in many courses for professionals (Reed and Procter, 1993; French *et al.*, 1994). The 'father' of these developments is generally acknowledged to be Donald Schön (1983, 1988) whose work has been mentioned in previous chapters and to which we shall return below. However, perhaps the first thing to be said about reflection in the context of thinking about the human relations of helping is that it is an integral part of day-to-day living. We all, some more than others, reflect on ourselves in relationships with others: 'Did I put my foot in it there?', 'What did she mean when she said . . . ?', 'What does he really think of me?' and so on and on. Reflection, in this sense, is central to our awareness of ourselves and our awareness of others. Also, reflection in this day-to-day sense is not a simple process but rather a tangle of knots, as in Laing's poem, which can bind and double-bind us in communication and relationships. This is because we are aware of the awareness of others. The nearest physical metaphor is a juxtaposition of mirrors in which reflections are endlessly reflected. Thus any of the questions posed above can be extended and extended: 'Did I put my foot in it?' can become, 'Does she know I think I put my foot in it?', which can become, 'I want her to think that I think that I put my foot in it' and so on and on.

This is not, as it might seem, a form of navel-gazing. It is pertinent to understanding Schön's notion of a reflective practitioner, or perhaps in this context, a 'reflective therapist'. He distinguishes in some detail between two models of theories-in-use or theories-in-action. Model I, sometimes called the traditional model, involves the following action strategies for the therapist: design and manage the environment so that the therapist is in control of the factors which he sees as relevant; own and control the task; unilaterally protect self by, for instance, withholding critical information; and unilaterally protect others, particularly the client, from being hurt. Schön associated this model with what he calls 'single loop' learning: 'Learning about strategies or tactics for achieving one's own objectives' (1988: 256). Model II, or the reflective practice model, is characterized by quite different action strategies: design situations in which all the participants, particularly the therapist and client, participate in defining and controlling relevant factors; the task is jointly controlled; protection of self is a joint enterprise, orientated towards growth; and bilateral protection of others.

Learning and development for therapists within model II is not a straight line of increased expertise in knowledge and skills. It is multi-faceted. It involves learning through experience, recognizing other perspectives, and working *with* rather than *on* people. It recognizes, too, that the dynamics of the human relations of helping and the integral processes of reflection are not esoteric to therapist–client relationships. They are best understood in terms of the general dynamics of human relations, that is, self-concepts, communication and relationships.

A crucial dimension of this model II perspective is the wider social and historical context. The ripples of understanding move outwards in ever increasing circles. For instance, to say that the therapist–client relationship is determined by the professional role of the therapist raises a whole series of questions about being a therapist:

1. How does each therapist adopt and adapt a professional role? What implications and meaning does this have for how therapists relate to clients?
2. How does any particular body of professionals define the professional role? What requirements, for instance, does a speech and language therapist have to fulfil in providing speech and language therapy?
3. Why and how has a particular body of professionals been established at this particular time and in this particular form? Why has a particular arena of expertise, such as knowledge and skills in speech and language therapy, been recognized as the domain and territory of one specific group of professionals, in this case speech and language therapists?

Personal reflections 10.1

There are a number of ways in which practitioners can engage in reflections. The following list is provided by Jill Reynolds (1992). You might have drawn on these modes of reflection if you have attempted the suggestions for 'Personal reflections'. As you read the list consider the following questions:

- which of these modes of reflection are open to you as a practitioner?
- which do you regularly engage in as a means of developing the human relations of helping as a therapist?
- which do you find helpful as a means of self development?

There are five possible modes of reflection, though the list is not exhaustive.

1. There are *conversations in the head*. As a therapist, you are continuously facing complex and ambiguous situations within which there are numerous possible interpretations and possibilities for action. Conversations in the head can review the possibilities, the judgements made and the criteria by which judgements are made.
2. *Informal conversations* can be a context for replaying events and experiences, with self-disclosure of thoughts and feelings.
3. *Written records* have played a major part in the suggestions for 'Personal reflections' in this book. Taped records might also be included here. The keeping of learning diaries (Bennett and Kingham, 1993) and journals (Fulwiler, 1987) is widely used as a part of courses for professionals which use a reflective practitioner type of approach.
4. The possibilities for discussions with a *partner*, who can act as a critical friend, is another mode of reflection which has been pursued in previous chapters.
5. Finally, there can be more formal arrangements for supervision or appraisal.

Discriminant reflections

Discriminant reflection focuses on the assessment of the effects of therapy. In the ideology of a market economy, questions of evaluation have become increasingly significant, at its simplest in a value-for-money sense, but also in far-reaching debates about the nature of therapy and the responsibilities of therapists. At Ashdown, a physiotherapist told us: 'What we want to develop in them is the motivation to try and tackle society, take it head on so that they can actually say "I want to go and do this, I want to go and do something else".' As we saw in Chapter 9, however, there was something of a struggle between professionals as to which type of therapy would best meet the client's needs, as defined by therapists, at any particular stage. A speech and language therapist told us:

> Say I'm helping a child with his eating and that improves his eating so he's able to feed himself, well that affects everything. It affects his relationships with his mum and anyone else that has had to feed him. It can give him self-esteem and more confidence to feel he's a capable person, more choice in what he eats and when he eats because he's in control. And that must be crucial.

The aims of therapy seem to be 'holistic', that is, concerned with the client as a whole person and every aspect of his life. Interventions into the client's life are justified on the grounds of being in the client's best interests. Teaching the client to be 'socially acceptable' can be justified under the guise of 'empowerment'.

So we return again to the problematic notion of 'empowerment'. A damning critique of the concept of empowerment comes from Gomm:

> Those people who say that they are in the business of empowering rarely seem to be giving up their own power; they are usually giving up someone else's and they may actually be increasing their own . . . the term 'empowerment' designates many excellent practices, and some dubious ones, but exactly what they are, and who is doing what to whom, is hidden by its usage. (1993: 137)

A counter-argument could suggest that the whole concept of empowerment as a giving away of power is simplistic. Empowerment can be seen as a joint concern with the empowerment of therapists being a joint enterprise with the empowerment of clients. Questions of empowerment are questions of the distribution of power: some individuals and groups have more say than others. They are also, however, about how power is used. To give an example, to be in a position of listening or not listening to another person is to be in a powerful position, and listening puts the other person in a powerful position in controlling what is talked about. If empowerment is the aim of therapy, then the challenge to therapists is to engage in a process of reflection which examines their roles in empowering clients. Taking empowerment as a central aim, by what criteria is the process of therapy to be judged?

Empowered therapist

Reflective practice can be directed towards the empowerment of both clients and therapists. As Osterman and Kottkamp argue,

> Reflective practice is an empowering and motivational process because it responds to basic human needs for competence, autonomy, and relatedness. The central reflective processes of communication and collaboration are empowering: they enable individuals to be more effective, to assume greater responsibility for their own performance, and to engage more closely and more productively with others in the workplace. (1993: 185)

A therapist who read an earlier draft of this book wrote about this in relation to her experiences keeping a journal:

> I've got into the habit of keeping a diary where I record the events of the day. I don't know that I'd call it a journal. At first it was a kind of unburdening, getting it off my chest so to speak. Now I've got into using it to think things through. I first of all put down what actually happened or my version of it anyway. Then I try to think of different possibilities. How other people might have seen it from their viewpoint: their views as I would

guess them. I then try to think of other things I might have done, how I might have approached it differently. It works as a kind of being wise after the event. . . . It has helped me. Not in the sense that I know all the answers now. In a way I'm stronger at saying I don't know all the answers. In fact, God preserve us from therapists that do think they know all the answers. It's helped me to be more flexible in my thinking, to see that there's always different answers, never a single right answer.

A reactive environment

A reactive environment is a social and physical environment which encourages and facilitates exploration of clients' understandings, feelings, preferences, desires and aspirations. The simplest form of choice-making, for instance, is an expression of preference. A reactive environment is one in which the expression of preferences is listened to, that is, 'listened' in its broadest sense. Thus, the use of counselling skills in therapy can help create a reactive environment. McInnes and Treffry (1982) have developed an approach to working with young people who are both deaf and blind which is founded upon the creation of a reactive rather than directive environment. They describe this as an environment which is characterized by social responsiveness based on emotional bonding, the establishment of close personal relationships and two-way communication. A specific example is the use of co-active techniques, which involve the therapist being immediately behind a child so that he has his back against the therapist's chest and the therapist can reach round to put his hands with the child's. In this way any activity, such as eating, can be undertaken moving together as one, rather than the therapist standing in front and feeding the child. Usually the therapist is in control at first but gradually encourages the child to take the lead.

Decision-making opportunities and skills

Choice as a decision-making process incorporates the expression of preferences but also involves active selection among alternatives. Choosing at this level, then, is an act based on decisions which may take into account not only preferences but also the perceived needs of others, perceived constraints and future goals. One key set of decisions and judgements is discriminant reflections themselves, that is to say any discussion of the effectiveness of therapy must include the clients' viewpoint. This was certainly not happening at Ashdown. The major concern seemed to be sharing such information with other professionals, as emphasized by one of the therapists:

> I think the most important thing is that we do establish with other professionals within the school a real understanding about what we are trying to achieve, an agreement and, as far as possible, a sharing of values between us as to what we are trying to achieve with these youngsters.

While such communication can be seen as important from the professionals' viewpoint, it will not necessarily be empowering for clients. It seems likely that it would be even more difficult to have any influence upon a team of professionals who have agreed the priorities than it would an individual professional working in isolation.

Advocacy

A focus on empowerment should look towards the collective, or group, as well as the individual. Simply in terms of your voice being heard, it is more powerful to speak on behalf of a collective voice as compared to your particular concerns as an individual. Ward and Mullender state:

> In groups personal troubles can be translated into common concerns. The experience of being with other people in the same boat can engender strength and new hope where apathy reigned beforehand: a sense of personal responsibility, internalized as self-blame, can find productive new outlets. It is for these reasons that it seems to us that groupwork lies at the heart of empowerment (1993: 153).

Personal reflections 10.2

Thinking of your work with a particular client or in general terms, answer the following questions in relation to discriminant reflections. They may make a good basis for discussions with a partner.

1. What criteria are important in evaluating your work as a therapist?
2. Who is directly involved in evaluating your work? If clients are involved, how are their views collected, recorded and taken into account in your work?
3. What evidence is collected and recorded to evaluate your work, such as direct observation, interviews and documentary evidence?
4. To what extent is empowerment part of the aims of your work as a therapist and how is this reflected in the criteria and processes used to evaluate your work?
5. Are the following taken into account in the evaluation of your work? If so, how?
   (a) empowered therapist
   (b) a reactive environment
   (c) decision-making opportunities and skills
   (d) advocacy.

Role reflections

Role reflections focus on the nature of therapy, the roles of the client and therapist and the therapist's and client's feelings, values and understandings in relation to their roles, including the constraints which determine therapist–client relationships. There are numerous restraints which can be seen as setting the boundaries on the human relations of helping in therapy, including: the length and frequency of contacts with clients; the degree of privacy for therapists working with clients; and as most often referred to by professionals at Ashdown, the very multi-professional system itself. Settings can differ considerably. Working in a Rehabilitation Centre, for instance, can involve frequent lengthy contacts with clients and other therapists, not only in therapy sessions but in corridors, sun lounges and so on, while working in a busy outpatient clinic can be quite different.

Time, or lack of it, seems to be the factor most often mentioned. An occupational therapist expressed the problems for her as follows: 'Time is the main factor. However much I would like to listen to the clients and respect their wishes, that takes time. It's not that simple. The more time I spend with one, the less time I have with others.' According to some therapists recent changes have added to the difficulties: '. . . increasing case loads and paperwork, and more patients at any one time, as well as managerial tasks such as audit and this will worsen as trusts become more in force.'

A major set of issues which have recurred throughout the discussions in this book related to the limitations imposed on human relation by roles, expectations and so on. Even the word 'professional' can have connotations of particular ways of acting and thinking which have implications in determining the relationship and communication between therapists and clients. Being professional is often seen in contrast to being informal, as in the therapist's construct grid in Chapter 1. Therapists, however, while adopting a professional role for themselves, can see themselves as working with clients as 'whole people' and everything about a client and his life might be delved into and opened up for the sake of therapy. In the research at Ashdown we found, for instance, that the professionals involved tended to see themselves as being concerned with the young people and their lives as a whole. This was complicated further by the fact that each professional also tended to see members of other professions as being restricted in their work and concerned with only limited aspects of young people and their lives. At its worst this is a laying bare of a client by a person doing her job in the best interests, as defined by the professional, of the client. Many disabled people see such intrusion as part of enforcing control over their lives and creating dependency: in other words intervention which creates rather than alleviates problems (Finkelstein, 1993).

What, then, of the use of counselling skills by therapists? Does this not promote a whole person approach? Certainly this is a danger which has been discussed a number of times in earlier chapters, for instance in the discussion of ethics (Chapter 2). There is, however, quite a different way of thinking about the whole person in helping, a way which is recognized in common phrases. If I say, for example, 'She treated me like a person', whether of a teacher, doctor, policewoman or dentist, it does not have the connotation that she delved into the intimate details of my life. On the contrary, it suggests that she treated me with respect and dignity and, perhaps above all, I felt a degree of control over the situation. It does not mean I had to answer every question the other person put to me, but rather that I could determine what was talked about from my side and, indeed, could remain silent if I wished, and my wishes were respected. It can also have the connotation of being two-way and mutual: she is acting as a person herself by treating me as a person. This is the whole person approach which has been developed and explored throughout this book. The first of the principles of helping, as listed in Table 4.1, is not only an aim for therapy, it applies to the process of therapy itself: 'To promote people's prediction and control over the decision-making processes which shape their lives.'

Personal reflections 10.3

Answer the following questions, thinking of your work with a particular client or in general terms. Your answers may make a good basis for discussions with a partner.

1. To what extent do you maintain a professional distance between yourself and your clients? Which aspects of you and your life do you feel are 'off-limits' to clients? Thinking of your work with a particular client: what aspects of yourself and your life did you feel able to talk about and which would you have never mentioned?
2. Think of your relationship with a particular client, if possible one you have written about in your journal. Make a list of the factors which affected, shaped or determined your relationship with this client, in particular those factors which are to do with the constraints of

working in your particular situation as a therapist. You might include such things as the length and frequency of contacts with the client. If it helps think of how your relationship with this client might have been different if, say, you had met him on holiday or he had moved in as your next door neighbour. Which of these factors you have named would you change, and how:

(a) to enable you to be yourself or more genuine in this relationship

(b) to promote greater mutuality and a more effective two-way flow of communication

(c) to enable the client to have more control over the process of therapy?

Judgemental reflections

Judgemental reflection is an awareness of your own values, likes and dislikes which you bring to bear in understanding and evaluating the process of therapy. As the research at Ashdown showed, people, in this instance professionals and parents, can differ considerably in their understanding of problems and solutions. The story of the multi-professional approach at the school is dominated by the struggle for power in defining problems and solutions. Brechin and Liddiard (1981) describe similar differences between the perceptions of professionals and disabled people. They report research using Kelly's construct grid in which people identified problems faced by disabled people and then used a triad approach (Chapter 1) to generate possible solutions. There were substantial differences between people's views. Daniel Rosen, for instance, was a 34-year-old disabled man living with his parents. The first five problems he identified were:

- not being able to go out when and where I want to
- not being able to get a proper job
- not being able to use public transport on my own
- not being able to mix with people of my own age
- not being able to mix with able-bodied people. (Brechin and Liddiard, 1981: 134)

The occupational therapist's list was quite different, to the extent that they could be talking about the problems of two different people:

- bathing
- not doing anything for himself – letting his parents do it
- deep-rooted psychological dependency on his parents
- lack of initiative for wanting to be independent
- was unable to put on a caliper. (1981: 136)

The possible solutions identified were, not surprisingly, also very different. The first three in Daniel's list were:

- having transport I could use
- knowing whether there are other people like me
- if people volunteered to give me lifts in their own cars. (1981: 134)

The first three in the occupational therapist's list were:

- something that has to be solved by long-term involvement of somebody who understands the problems and can set objectives
- something that cannot be solved
- introduction of the idea of something different to what he's used to. (1981: 136)

The general findings of the research reported by Brechin and Liddiard (1981) reflect Daniel Rosen's specific case. Professionals tend to define problems in terms of the individual: dysfunction, lack of skills, lack of motivation, inability to undertake particular activities and so on. Disabled people, on the other hand, tend to define their own problems in social terms: lack of opportunities, barriers to access, segregation and so on.

Personal reflections 10.4

This exercise is an adapted version of the research reported by Brechin and Liddiard (1981). Its aim is to explore and think about possible differences in judgements between yourself as a therapist and your clients. It uses the construct grid which was introduced in Chapter 1. The steps are as follows:

1. Select a client with whom to do this exercise.
2. Make a list of the problems the client has faced and still faces.
3. Use this list of problems to think about the possible solutions. Consider the problems in groups of three and suggest how two are the same and one is different in terms of solutions. For example, Daniel Rosen's occupational therapist might have looked at the combination of the first three problems in her list: '1. Bathing; 2. Not doing anything for himself – letting his parents do it; and 3. Deep-rooted psychological dependency on his parents.' A possible solution for the last two but not the first is: 'Something that has to be solved by long-term involvement of somebody who understands the problems and can set objectives.'
4. This is repeated using different combinations of three problems until a list of possible solutions has been identified.
5. Finally consider each problem from your list in turn and identify any of the possible solutions which might apply to it. In this way you will get an indication of how you understand problems. For Daniel Rosen's occupational therapist, for instance, 'bathing' is not a problem relating to long-term training. Her construct grid suggests she related bathing to what she saw as Daniel's lack of motivation and the use of aids, in particular a bath board.
6. Now go through the same procedure helping the client to identify his problems and possible solutions from his viewpoint. This is best done by giving the client sufficient instructions so that he can go through the exercise on his own. It can be done by interviewing the client, but great care needs to be taken not to distort his views.
7. The final step is to share and discuss both analyses of problems and solutions with the client concerned. Where do the similarities and differences lie?

Conceptual reflections

Conceptual reflection involves an awareness of the constructs which you use in understanding and evaluating yourself in your role as therapist. There are many struggles over language and meaning which are crucial to the work of therapists. There are concepts which are used to refer to people receiving therapy: 'patients', 'clients', 'users' and so on. Indeed recent changes in the use of terminology have involved connotations that the person receiving therapy is being given more respect and even more control over the therapy they receive. Oliver is sceptical, however:

> The professional–client relationship can itself also be dependency creating, and indeed the very language used suggests that power is unequally distributed within this relationship. Recent attempts to address this problem through changing the terminology from 'client' to 'user' or customer', acknowledge that the problem exists but do little to change the structures within which these power relations are located. (1989: 13–14)

Though changes in terminology do not necessarily have significant effects on relationships and processes of help, there are real conflicts over the meaning of terms which do have far-reaching implication for understanding the whole process of therapy. Arguments over definitions are often reduced to supposedly technical purposes, but they are in effect part of the struggle to establish and legitimize one way of thinking over another. They are 'battles for the mind' which have implications for who receives help, who provides help and what help is provided.

The idea of 'struggle' is important here. This is not an academic exercise to show that there are different interpretations, different ideas of what help is required. This is not a game played by neutral observers. These are real struggles between individuals and between groups, and such struggles are played out in the direct helper–helped relationship. Politicians, managers, accountants and so on are all also involved in these struggles, and crucial to this idea of struggle is that not everyone is equal in the process of authorizing help.

The idea of a 'struggle of voices', which was introduced in the previous chapter, has a number of crucial elements:

1. Individuals and groups have their own perspectives which give meaning to themselves, their situation, their experiences and their social world.
2. Individuals and groups create, develop and change meanings throughout their everyday interactions with each other.
3. Individuals and groups are not passive in the processes of social construction. Each arrives at an interpretation of reality, his 'truths', which suit his own interests and then deploys and promotes his interpretations of events, trying to convert others to his way of understanding.
4. There is a distribution of control or power between participants in day-to-day struggles. Some people have more power than others to influence 'reality construction', and participate in the decision-making which shapes their lives.

A major theme of the research at Ashdown centred upon the definition or, more broadly, the meaning of disability. Though discussed explicitly at times, this was more defuse as a topic and ran inherently through a wide range of concerns. In essence, disability was consistently viewed as a condition of the individual. Sometimes this was stated explicitly, as by a physiotherapist:

> I look on the disability as being the overall diagnosis . . . to me the children have got a disability i.e. spina bifida, cerebral palsy to me that's the disability. That's the underlying problem. . . .

Others were more circumspect. The doctor, for instance, stated:

> I use the World Health Organisation classification of impairment, disability and handicap, and handicap is the social effect of the disadvantage suffered because of a person having disability which means a loss or an alteration of function due to impairment.

It is still clearly evident from this classification that the individual young person is the source of the problem. This is an 'individual model' of disability.

As we saw in Chapter 4, disabled people have been advocating a totally different definition of disability. Mike Oliver summarized this stance as follows:

> All disabled people experience disability as social restriction, whether those restrictions occur as a consequence of inaccessible environments, questionable notions of intelligence and social competence, the inability of the general population to use sign language, the lack of reading material in braille or hostile public attitudes to people with non-visible disabilities (Oliver, 1990: xiv).

From the viewpoint of disabled people, disability is imposed on people by disabling barriers: it is not a condition of the individual. Some professional definitions, for instance the so-called 'socio-medical approach' have attempted to take a broader social perspective. Yet the perspective remains focused on the individual in statements such as: 'We need a socio-medical approach that incorporates the medical and social perspectives in assessing, preventing, and caring for people with disabling conditions' (Patrick, 1989: 2). Such definitions are generated by the needs of professionals, not disabled people. From the viewpoint of disabled people, the focus becomes the barriers faced in a society geared by and for non-disabled people – barriers which exclude disabled people from full active citizenship. This is often referred to as a social model of disability and can be conveyed as a cycle of repression, as in Figure 10.1.

The crucial factor in breaking this cycle is the control by disabled people of their own lives and a say in their community. Disability, and how it is overcome, is defined by disabled people: their understandings, their intentions and desires. The transformation of power relations is fundamental to overcoming disabling barriers and establishing enabling environments. This involves the establishment of equal opportunities and support for the emancipation of oppressed groups within society.

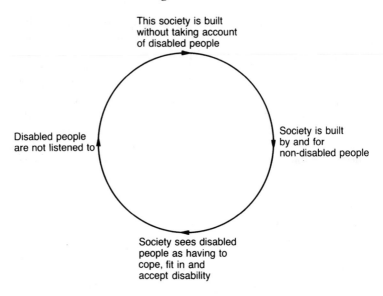

Figure 10.1   *Disabling circle*

Personal reflections 10.5

This exercise has been adapted from Finkelstein (1980).

1. Make a list of adjectives or phrases which describe the way you see disabled people *in general.*
2. Next to each of the adjectives or phrases write what you consider to be its opposite 'pole'.
3. The list of bipolar constructs you have generated can help you in thinking about how you see disabled in relation to non-disabled people. Which of your constructs suggests that you have an individual model of disability and which suggests a social model.
4. What direct implications do these two different models have for working with disabled people?

Theoretical reflections

Theoretical reflection is an awareness of how your own values and constructs are based upon taken for granted and culturally embedded assumptions about the nature of what we are as human beings, the nature of human relations, the processes of helping and the processes of therapy. The following are two major themes, in the form of questions, which arose in the research at Ashdown. They pertain to core issues for therapists in the human relationships of helping through therapy: the two-way flow of communication and mutuality in the therapist-client relationship.

- Helpful relationships in which the decisions of others are imposed on disabled people or relationships which enable young people to have a greater say in their own lives?.

There are, then, real dilemmas for those who want to help young disabled people. On one hand, it can seem that there are certain ways in which young people can be helped: regimens they should follow; treatments that are essential to their well-being; skills and knowledge they require; and risks from which they need to be sheltered. Such forms of help are seen as enabling young people, in the long term, to have control over their own lives. Two therapists, a senior speech and language therapist and a senior physiotherapist working in a Regional Rehabilitation Centre, commented: 'People come to therapy with the expectation to be treated and cured. Would they feel uncertain if this was not tackled directly as it is done presently?'

On the other hand, relationships which impose such forms of help, encourage apathy and passivity on the part of young disabled people. Young people learn that decisions are made by others and they learn to be controlled. So even in later years when opportunities might arise for young disabled people to have some choices and to have more say, they have no basis for such autonomy. Young people can be helped to be helpless. A disabled woman describing the impact of her repeated hospitalizations as a child writes:

In all my hospital experiences, the saddest part was always the same. All those people trying so hard to help me: the nurses, the doctors, the volunteers, the Shriners. All of them hoping for me to get better and do well, all wanting to be kind and useful, all feeling how important helping me was, yet never did any one of them ask me what it was like for me. They never asked me what I wanted for myself. They never asked me if I wanted their help. (Saxton, 1988: 55)

This denial of control over the processes of help by the receivers of help can take many forms. For some disabled people, for instance, the pressures to be normal and independent in non-disabled people's terms include discouragement from asking for any help.

- A team which determines the lives of others, or democratic participation in decision-making for all?

As in the provision of services for disabled people generally, Ashdown School consists of a number of professional groups each with its own ways of working, and its own viewpoints and responsibilities. This system is itself a source of many difficulties for professionals and parents: some practical, some personal and some organizational. How is this whole organization seen in relation to the decision-making that shapes young disabled people's lives, and in particular the say that they themselves have? On the one hand there is a widely held concern to improve the effectiveness of professionals working together, and involving parents, to create a system in which there is openness, effective communication and negotiated decisions about priorities for young disabled people. On the other hand, the system itself denies young people opportunities and circumstances in which they can have control over their own lives. The system itself creates dependency in that young people are passed from the hands of one professional to another, pressurized by the demands of each professional discipline and have their 'needs' determined by others.

The two therapists commented that the system also does not facilitate a concern for human relations on the part of therapists: 'We work in a multi-disciplinary team of approximately five therapists. If we all try to take the role of counsellor, it would be too much for the patient. . . . Will therapists feel inadequate if a client has opened up to another therapist and not them?'

The two therapists wrote:

Our willingness to reflect on ourselves and to challenge *our* assumptions and prejudices is essential to learning to use counselling skills. This in itself requires courage and effort on the part of the therapist and may require help from additional people. People often fear what they may find in themselves. . . . Therapists need support to help them become more self-aware. They cannot be expected to do it all alone and facilities are very *rarely* available therefore put up a brick wall. . . . With the introduction of teams, it is becoming easier to cope and support each other, plan strategies and allow helping to continue, especially when a particularly stressful client is admitted.

But the last word goes to a disabled woman who shares with us a challenging view of disability (Meredith, 1994: 105):

Are you **D**eaf?
Are you bl**I**nd?
  Can't you **S**ee me?
  Can't you he**A**r me?
    And do you **B**lame
      my disab**I**lity
        for your **L**ack
          of ins**I**ght,
          for your shor**T**comings?
            Do **Y**ou?

References

Argyle, M. and Henderson, M. (1985) *The Anatomy of Relationships*, Penguin Books, Harmondsworth

Atkinson, D. and Ward, L. (1986) *Strategies for Change*, Book 4 of the course (P555) 'Mental Handicap: Patterns for Living', Open University Press, Milton Keynes

Bell, J. (1987) *Doing Your Research Project*, Open University Press, Milton Keynes

Bennett, J. and Kingham, M. (1993) Learning diaries. In Reed, J. and Procter, S. (eds), *Nurse Education: A Reflective Approach*, Edward Arnold, London

Bennett, P. (1993) *Counselling for Heart Disease*, British Psychological Society Books, Leicester

Bolton, R. (1979) *People Skills: How to Assert, Listen and Resolve Conflict*, Prentice-Hall, Englewood Cliffs, New Jersey

Bond, T. (1993) Counselling, counselling skills and professional roles. In Bayne, R. and Nicolson, P. (eds.), *Counselling and Psychology for Health Professionals*, Chapman and Hall, London

Braude M. (ed.) (1987) *Women, Power and Therapy*, Haworth Press, New York

Brechin, A. and Liddiard, P. (1981) *Look at it This Way: New Perspectives in Rehabilitation*, Hodder and Stoughton, Sevenoaks

Brechin, A. and Swain, J. (1987) *Changing Relationships*, Harper and Row, London

Brechin, A. and Swain, J. (1988) Professional/client relationships: creating a 'working allience' with people with learning difficulties. *Disability, Handicap and Society*, **3**(3), 213–226

British Association of Counselling (1994) *Invitation to Membership*, British Association of Counselling, Rugby

Burgoon, M., Hunsaker, F.G. and Dawson, E.J. (1994) *Human Communication*, 3rd edn, Sage, London

Burnard, P. (1989) *Counselling Skills for Health Professionals*, Chapman and Hall, London

Burnard, P. (1990) *Learning Human Skills: An Experiential Guide for Nurses* (2nd edn), Butterworth-Heinemann, Oxford

Burnard, P. (1992) *Know Yourself! Self-Awareness Activities for Nurses*, Scutari Press, London

Burnard, P. (1994) *Counselling Skills for Health Professionals*, (2nd edn), Chapman and Hall, London

Carroll, L. (1923) *Alice's Adventures in Wonderland*, George Allen and Unwin, London

Chaplin, J. (1988) *Feminist Counselling in Action*, Sage, London

Churchill, L. (1977) Ethical issues of a professional in transition. *American Journal of Nursing*, **77**(5) 873–875

Cohn, E.S. (1983) Effects of victims' and helpers' attributions for problem and solution on reactions to receiving help. In Nadler, A., Fisher, J.D. and DePaulo, B.M. (eds), *New Directions in Helping*, Vol. 3, Academic Press, London

Cooley, C.H. (1902) *Human Nature and the Social Order*, Scribner's, New York

Cooper, C. (1984) Psychodynamic therapy: the Kleinian approach. In Dryden, W. (ed.), *Individual Therapy in Britain*, Harper and Row, London

Coopersmith, S. (1967) *The Antecedents of Self-Esteem*, Freeman, San Francisco

Corey, M.S. and Corey, G. (1993) *Becoming a Helper*, 2nd edn, Brooks/Cole, Pacific Grove, California

Corker, M. (1994) *Counselling– The Deaf Challenging*, Jessica Kingsley, London

Coupe, J., Barber, M. and Murphy, D. (1988) Affective Communication. In Coupe, J. and Goldbart, J. (eds),

Communication Before Speech: Normal Development and Impaired Communication, Croom Helm, London

Crompton, M. (1992) *Children and Counselling*, Edward Arnold, London

Culley, S. (1990) *Integrative Skills in Action*, Sage, London

Dalton, P. (1994) *Counselling People with Communication Problems*, Sage, London

Davis, H. (1993) *Counselling Parents of Children with Chronic Illness or Disability*, British Psychological Society Books, Leicester

Davis, H. and Fallowfield, L. (1991) Counselling and communication in health care: the current situation. In Davis, H. and Fallowfield, L. (eds), *Counselling and Communication in Health Care*, Wiley, Chichester

Derlega, V.J., Metts, S., Petronio, S. and Margulis, S.T. (1993) *Self-Disclosure*, Sage, London

Dewey, J. (1933) *How We Think: A Restatement of the Relation of Reflective Thinking to the Educative Process*, Henry Regnery, Chicago

Dickson, D.A., Hargie, O.D.W. and Morrow, N.C. (1989) *Communication Skills Training for Health Professionals: An Instructor's Handbook*, Chapman and Hall, London

Dominelli, L. (1990) *Women and Community Action*, Venture Press, Birmingham

Doyal, L. and Gough, I. (1991) *A Theory of Human Need*, Macmillan, Basingstoke

Drauker, C.B. (1992) *Counselling Survivors of Childhood Sexual Abuse*, Sage, London

Dryden, W. (ed). (1984) *Individual Therapy in Britain*, Harper and Row, London

Egan, G. (1977) *You and Me: The skills of communicating and relating to others*, Brooks/Cole, Pacific Grove, California

Egan, G. (1990) *The Skilled Helper: Model, Skills and Methods for Effective Helping*, 4th edn, Brooks/Cole, Monterey

Finkelstein, V. (1980) *Know Your Own Approach*, P251, Block 2, Unit 4, Open University Press, Milton Keynes

Finkelstein, V. (1993) Disability: a social challenge or an administrative responsibility? In Swain, J., Finkelstein, V., French, S. and Oliver, M. (eds), *Disabling Barriers– Enabling Environments*, Sage, London

Flynn, N. and Common, R. (1992) *Contracting For Care*, The Joseph Rowntree Foundation, York

Foucault, M. (1986) An Interview with Michel Foucault. In Charles Raus (tr.), *Death and the Labyrinth: The World of Michel Foucault*, Athlone Press, London

Fransella, F. and Dalton, P. (1990) *Personal Construct Counselling in Action*, Sage, London

French, S. (1992) Clinical interviewing. In French, S. (ed.), *Physiotherapy: A Psychosocial Approach*, Butterworth–Heinemann, Oxford

French, S. (1993) *Practical Research: A Guide for Therapists*, Butterworth–Heinemann, Oxford

French, S., Neville, S. and Laing, J. (1994) *Teaching and Learning: A Guide for Therapists*, Butterworth–Heinemann, Oxford

Fulwiler, T. (ed.) (1987) *The Journal Book*, Boynton/Cook, Portsmouth, New Hampshire

Gazda, G.M., Asbury, F.R., Balzer, F.J. *et al.* (1977) *Human Relations Development: A Manual for Educators*, 2nd edn, Allyn and Bacon, Inc., Boston

Gomm, R. (1993) Issues of power in health and welfare. In Walmsley, J., Reynolds, J., Shakespeare, P. and Woolfe, R. (eds), *Health, Welfare and Practice: Reflecting on Roles and Relationships*, Sage, in association with The Open University, London

Hall, E. and Hall, C. (1988) *Human Relations in Education*, Routledge, London

Harris, T. (1973) *I'm OK, You're OK*, Pan, London

Hewitt, J.P. (1984) *Self and Society: A Symbolic Interactionist Social Psychology*, 3rd edn, Allyn and Bacon, Inc., Boston

Jacobs, M. (1988) *Psychodynamic Counselling in Action*, Sage, London

Jung, C.C. (1964) *Man and his Symbols*, Aldus Books, London

Jung, C.C. (1978) *Selected Writings*, Fontana, London

Kanfer, F.H. and Goldstein, A.P. (eds), (1980) *Helping People Change: A Textbook of Methods*, 2nd edn, Pergamon, New York

Karuza, J., Zeven, M.A., Rabinowitz, V. and Brickman, P. (1982) Attribution of responsibility by helpers and recipients. In Wills, T.A. (ed.) *Basic Processes in Helping Relationships*, Academic Press, London

Kelly, G.A. (1955) *The Psychology of Personal Constructs*, Norton, New York

Kottler, J.A. and Kottler, E. (1993) *Teacher as Counselor: Developing the Healing Skills You Need*, Corwin Press, Newbury Park

Laing, R.D. (1970) *Knots*, Tavistock Publications, London

Larkin, P. (1988) *Collected Poems*, The Marvell Press and Faber and Faber, London

Ley, P. (1988) *Communicating with Patients: Improving Communication, Satisfaction and Compliance*, Croom Helm, London

Luft, J. (1969) *Of Human Interaction: The Johari Model*, Mayfield, Palo Alto

Macchielli, R. (1983) *Face to Face in the Counselling Interview*, Macmillan Press, London

MacLean, D. and Gould, S. (1988) *The Helping Process: An Introduction*, Croom Helm, London

MacWhannell, D. E. (1992) Communication in physiotherapy practice. In French, S. (ed.) *Physiotherapy: A Psychosocial Approach*, Butterworth–Heinemann, Oxford

Marková, I. (1987) *Human Awareness: Its Social Development*, Hutchinson, London

Marsh, P. and Fisher, M. (1992) *Good Intentions: Developing Partnership in Social Services*, Joseph Rowntree Foundation, York

Maslow, A. (1954) *Motivation and Personality*, 2nd edn, Harper and Row, York

Mayo, E. (1933) *The Human Problems of an Industrial Civilization*, Macmillan, New York

McInnes, J.M. and Treffry, J.A. (1982) *Deaf-Blind Infants and Children: A Developmental Guide*, Open University Press, Milton Keynes

McKnight, J. (1977) Professionalised service and disabling help. In Illich, I. (ed.), *Disabling Professions*, Marion Boyars, London

McLeod, J. (1993) *An Introduction to Counselling*, Open University Press, Buckingham

Mearns, D. and Thorne, B. (1988) *Person-Centred Counselling in Action*, Sage, London

Meredith, J. (1994) Disability. In Keith, L. (ed.), *Mustn't Grumble: Writing by Disabled Women*, The Women's Press, London

Morris, J. (1991) *Pride Against Prejudice*, Women's Press, London

Munro, E.A., Manthei, R.J. and Small, J.J. (1983) *Counselling: A Skills Approach*, revised edition, Methuen, Auckland, New Zealand

Murgatroyd, S. (1985) *Counselling and Helping*, British Psychological Society/Methuen, London

Nelson-Jones, R. (1982) *The Theory and Practice of Counselling Psychology*, Holt, Rinehart and Winston, London

Nelson-Jones, R. (1986) *Human Relations Skills*, Holt, Rinehart and Winston, London

Oliver, M. (1989) Disability and dependency: a creation of industrial societies. In Barton, L. (ed.) *Disability and Dependency*, Falmer Press, Lewes

Oliver, M. (1990) *The Politics of Disablement*, Macmillan, London

Oliver, M. (1993) *Disability, Citizenship and Empowerment*, Workbook 2 of the course (K665) 'The Disabling Society', Open University Press, Milton Keynes

Osterman, K. F. and Kottkamp, R. B. (1993) *Reflective Practice for Educators: Improving Schooling Through Professional Development*, Corwin Press, Newbury Park, California

Parry, A. (1985) *Physiotherapy Assessment*, 2nd edn, Chapman and Hall, London

Patrick, D.L. (1989) A socio-medical approach to disablement. In Patrick, D.L. and Peach, H. (eds), *Disablement in the Community*, Oxford University Press, Oxford

Penman, R. (1980) *Communication Processes and Relationships*, Academic Press, London

Reed, J. and Procter, S. (eds) (1993) *Nurse Education: A Reflective Approach*, Edward Arnold, London

Rees, S. and Graham, R.S. (1991) *Assertion Training: How to be Who You Really Are*, Tavistock/Routledge, London

Reynolds, J. and Dimmock, B. (1992) *Theory and Practice Part 2: Reflection in Practice*, Workbook 3 of the course (K663) 'Roles and Relationships', Open University Press, Milton Keynes

Rogers, C.R. (1957) The necessary and sufficient conditions of therapeutic personality change. *Journal of Consulting Psychology*, **21**, 95–103

Rogers, C.R. (1961) *On Becoming a Person*, Houghton Mifflin, Boston

Rogers, C.R. (1978) *Carl Rogers on Personal Power: Inner Strength and its Revolutionary Impact*, Constable, London

Rogers, C.R. (1980) *A Way of Being*, Houghton Mifflin, Boston

Rogers, C.R. (1983) *Freedom to Learn for the 80s*, Charles E. Merrill, Columbus

Rogers, C.R. and Stevens, B. (1967) *Person to Person: The Problem of being Human*, Real People Press, Layfayette, California

Ross, A.O. (1992) *The Sense of Self: Research and Theory*, Springer, New York

Rowan, J. (1983) *The Reality Game: A Guide to Humanistic Counselling and Therapy*, Routledge and Kegan Paul, London

Russell, R. and Laing, R.D. (1992) *R.D. Laing and Me: Lessons in Love*, Hillgarth Press, New York

Saxton, M. (1988) The something that happened before I was born. In Saxton, M. and Howe, F. (eds) *With Wings: An Anthology of Literature by Women with Disabilities*, Virago Press, London

Schön, D. (1983) *The Reflective Practitioner*, Basic Books, New York

Schön, D. (1988) *Educating the Reflective Practitioner*, Jossey-Bass, San Francisco

Searle, J. (1976) A classification of illocutionary acts. *Language in Society*, **5**, 1–23

Segal, J. (1993) Against self-disclosure. In Dryden, W. (ed.), *Questions and Answers on Counselling in Action*, Sage, London

Sim, J. (1992) Ethical decision-making in physiotherapy. In French, S. (ed.), *Physiotherapy: A Psychosocial Approach*, Butterworth–Heinemann, Oxford

Skinner, B.F. (1953) *Science and Human Behaviour*, Macmillan, New York

Sullivan, A. (1994) Part of a Life. In Keith, L. (ed.), *Mustn't Grumble: Writing by Disabled Women*, The Women's Press, London

Swain, J., Finkelstein, V., French, S. and Oliver, M. (eds) (1993) *Disabling Barriers: Enabling Environments*, Sage, London

Thomas, P. (1991) A therapeutic journey through the garden of Eden. *Counselling*, November, 143–154

Thompson, S.B.N. and Morgan, M. (1990) *Occupational Therapy for Stroke Rehabilitation*, Chapman and Hall, London

Tolstoy, L. (1954) *Anna Karenin*, Penguin Books, Harmondsworth

Torrington, D. (1982) *Face to Face in Management*, Prentice-Hall, Englewood Cliffs, New Jersey

Trower, P., Bryant, B. and Argyle, M. (1978) *Social Skills and Mental Health*, Methuen, London

Trower, P., Casey, A. and Dryden, W. (1988) *Cognitive-Behavioural Counselling in Action*, Sage, London

Tschudin, V. (1991) *Counselling Skills for Nurses*, 3rd edn, Baillière Tindall, London

Ward, D. and Mullender, A. (1993) Empowerment and oppression: an indissoluable pairing for contemporary social work. In Walmsley, J., Reynolds, J., Shakespeare, P. and Woolfe, R. (eds), *Health, Welfare and Practice: Reflecting on Roles and Relationships*, Sage in association with The Open University, London

Watzlawick, P., Bearin, J.H. and Jackson, D.D. (1967) *Pragmatics of Human Communication*, Norton, New York

Williams, J. (1993) What is a profession? Experience versus expertise. In Walmsley, J., Reynolds, J., Shakespeare, P. and Woolfe, R. (eds), *Health, Welfare and Practice: Reflecting on Roles and Relationships*, Sage in association with The Open University, London

Woody, R.H., Hansen, J.C. and Rossberg, R.H. (1989) *Counseling Psychology: Strategies and Services*, Brooks/Cole, Pacific Grove, California

Index